Ocean of Stre-

*This book is dedicated
to the beloved memory
of my mother
Susan Blaney Wilkinson*

Ocean of Streams

Second Revised Edition

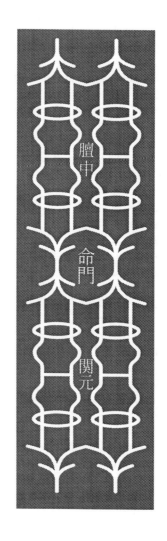

膻中

命門

関元

Zen Shiatsu
Meridians, Tsubos and Theoretical Impressions

Veet Allan

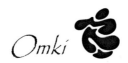

Omki

Hello Aurelius, Chang and Gorak!

Text, cover design and illustrations by Veet Allan

Copyright © 2006 and 2007 by Veet Allan

Title first published in 1994 by Om Shiatsu Centre

This edition published by Omki
Morton Holm Cottage, Keir Mill,
Thornhill, DG3 4DQ, Scotland UK

First Edition, August 1994
ISBN-10: 0-9523976-0-9
Reprinted 1995
Reprinted 1996
Reprinted 1997
Reprinted 1998
Roprinted 2000 (with additional illustrations)
Reprinted 2003

Second Edition, May 2006
Revised, June 2007
ISBN-10: 0-9523976-2-5
ISBN-13: 978-0-9523976-2-5

www.omki.co.uk
e-mail: info@omki.co.uk

This book is not designed to diagnose, prescribe, or treat any ailment without adequate professional training or supervision. It is therefore not intended in any way as a replacement for proper medical consultation. Any uses of the contents of this publication are the responsibility of the reader.

Contents ━━━━━━━━━━

Preface

When the original edition of this book was published in 1994, my goal was to present an accessible and detailed illustrated textbook for students based on the curriculum of the Shiatsu Society in this country. I never imagined back then, that it would be so well received and used by students and practitioners worldwide, let alone that I would be writing the preface to a second edition now, twelve years later and subsequently one year on, revising it.

Initially, I saw the original Zen Shiatsu meridian chart, by the late Japanese master Shizuto Masunaga, in 1980 at several introductory Shiatsu workshops held in Glasgow, by Anima, a Japanese female graduate of his Iokai school in Tokyo. However, I could never really comprehend Masunagas system until 1989-91, when I had the good fortune to study with Pauline Sasaki and Clifford Andrews at three of their annual springtime residentials held in England. Their clear teaching, guidance and development of the original Masunaga system was simply a revelation at the time.

Shortly after this period. I attended a workshop with Shinmei Kishi in London. Kishi was an early student of Shizuto Masunagas in Japan and had also tutored Pauline Sasaki. During a treatment from Kishi I experienced flashes of thunder, gold colour and lightning. The Kishi method was something different, not meridians other things! In recollection I am most fond of a moment when Nick Pole, a teacher with the Shiatsu college asked Kishi "What about the Zen Shiatsu meridian chart?" to which he replied "ask Masunaga!" From that moment the road was open.

As a Shiatsu practitioner I began to use and travel the Masunaga meridian routes regularly in my practice. Subsequently, as a teacher presenting illustrations to my students I found myself adjusting their routes in accordance with my experience in practice and my then theoretical understanding of them. This material was published as 'Ocean of Streams' in 1994.

For a further Nine years I continued to explore, revise and expand this Zen Shiatsu based meridian system. The initial expansion of this process came by way of intuition, spontaneous execution of technique and spiritual guidance. However, in order to research this evolving map and look at the roots of the Shizuto Masunaga system I began to read English translations of the Chinese medical classics. Particularly, the 'Systematic Classic of Acupuncture and Moxibustion' (Zhen Jiu Jia Yi Jing 針灸甲乙經), the 'Spiritual Pivot' (Ling Shu 靈樞), the 'Simple Questions' (Su Wen 素問), the 'Classic of Difficulties' (Nan Jing 難經) and notably, the various commentaries on the classics and

studies of Chinese medical characters by Cluade Larre and Elisabeth Rochat de la Vallée, in their excellent series of books entitled 'Chinese Medicine from the Classics'.

From these studies and that of various modern Acupuncture texts I soon found myself adapting and illustrating for Shiatsu treatment, full body charts (unpublished to date) of the Zen Shiatsu meridians and Classical Chinese channels, with their various divergencies in one set and the Extraordinary vessels in another.

With regard to the translation of the channel / meridian and vessel names. I have adopted those found in the works of Paul U.Unschuld, Claude Larre and Elizabeth Rochat de la Vallée, that have gelled with my experience to date. Please note that the Chinese term or word Qi (氣), is romanised as Ki throughout all the Japanese influenced Zen Shiatsu sections. In differentiating the various teaching approaches the term Jing (經) is translated here as 'channel' throughout the Classical Chinese sections, whereas 'meridian' is preferred for the Zen Shiatsu sections. Naturally, the reader or student may still prefer to substitute these with other standards or abbreviations that they are already familiar with.

I found the process of digesting the technical complexities of the various systems rather unpalatable at first. However, in time I realised that most of what I considered to be 'new lightways' or meridians were mostly there all along, just categorised differently with regard to Classical Chinese Acupuncture and Shizuto Masunaga's Japanese styled Shiatsu. The basic mapping of the aforementioned systems was completed in 2004, by which time I had stopped practicing and teaching Shiatsu completely, in favour of the art of drawing and illustration. Thankfully, some of the Zen Shiatsu based work is made available here, for the first time.

It is therefore, with a great sense of gratitude and satisfaction that I present this second edition, expanded, revised and completely re-illustrated using modern digital illustration techniques. My hope and prayer is that this book will continue to be a useful resource for all students and practitioners of Oriental medicine, and enlighten their own perceptions and treatment of the meridians for the supreme health and benefit of all.

Veet Allan
Thornhill
2006
rev. 2007

Acknowledgements

Namaste,

Jila-Elizabeth, Suzanne, Denise,
Erin, Déva, Kieran and Elle Beth

Hearty thanks to all my clients, students and teachers who have
contributed to and shaped my experience in Shiatsu and Oriental medicine.

Remembered again, the Anima Yuan.

Gratitude to the three treasures for the vital spark....
Clifford Andrews, Pauline Sasaki and Shinmei Kishi.

Special vibes to the following for their timely support
and encouragement towards this edition.

Acumedic Ltd (England), Liz Arundel, Bertram Books (England),
Katrina Billings, Patricia E. Carusone (USA), China Books (Australia),
Oliver Cowmeadow, Simon Fall, Suzanne Franzen,
Gardners Books (England), Shruti Gordon, Tamsin Grainger,
Kris Larthe, Jane Martin, Janet McDonald,
Ina Neuner (Germany), Bill Palmer, Keith Philips, Ray Ridolfi
Nicola Pooley, Ulrike Schmidt (Germany) and Kate Turner.

Finally, thanks to everyone worldwide who purchased
the original book and this current edition.
For it is you after all, that have ensured it still remains in print today.

Layout and Colouring Guide

This book contains ten main chapters plus an appendix, bibliography, glossary of Chinese terms, point (residential tsubo) names glossary and point indications index.

Chapter One presents a basic outline of the Oriental measurement system for the Human body. This is then augmented with fully annotated illustrations of the skeletal, muscular and organ systems of Western medicine.

Chapter Two contains various tables and illustrations of Diagnostic information from Classical Chinese medicine including Yin-Yang, the Five elements, the vital substances, face, tongue, pulse, the shu and mu points. The chapter concludes with illustrations of the standard Zen Shiatsu hara (abdominal) and back diagnostic areas, the basic Kyo-Jitsu modes and Tsubo types plus the Zen Shiatsu meridian/germ layer functions.

Chapter Three is based on two of the Primary (extraordinary) vessels) namely the Du mai (Supervisor vessel) and the Ren mai (Controller vessel). Contents include Classical point (residential tsubo) studies, vessel correspondences and fully annotated illustrations of the above vessels.

Chapters Four through to Nine are headed by one of the Five elements or phases from Classical Chinese medicine in sequence beginning with Water, then Wood, Fire (over two chapters), then Earth and concluding with Metal. Each chapter is then subdivided to contain the relevant Classical point (residential tsubo) studies, Zang Fu (organ)/Zen Shiatsu (meridian) functions, Five element and Zen Shiatsu meridian correspondences. Fully annotated illustrations of the relevant Zen Shiatsu based meridians conclude each chapter.

Chapter Ten contains a fully illustrated study of all the Zen Shiatsu based meridians in key body areas or zones. These are augmented with anatomical cross sections, which should be viewed and interpreted as looking from below the body and upwards towards the head.

The book concludes with the following. An appendix containing the author's alternative Zen Shiatsu based diagnostic schema for the body. Including the head, neck, chest, back and hara (abdominal) zones. A bibliography. A glossary of Chinese medical terms including the points and meridians. All categorised according to Western notation, romanised name, Chinese character and pinyin name. A points indications index according to Western medical indications, referenced to the page number the relevant point or points studies appear in.

All illustrations and tables including the Five element symbols, are designed for self-colouring. To obtain the best results for the meridian illustrations, use good quality coloured fine felt pens. However, you may prefer to use coloured pencils for safe completion of the initial layout. Then later, highlight the meridians with fine felt-tip pens to present a more luminous detail against the original shaded anatomy. All other illustrations and tables are best shaded with coloured pencils as you prefer.

The colour for each meridian is related to its associated element and is further differentiated into lighter or darker shades according to their Yin or Yang status respectfully. The points or tsubos are better left uncoloured as this helps boost the overall clarity of the illustrations. A full legend (opposite) is provided as a guide for self colouring and referencing.

To preserve the quality of the drawings and prevent bleed from felt tip pens or indentation from coloured pencils it is suggested that you insert a thicker page or card directly behind the page you are colouring.

Colour Legend and Reference

Symbol	Meridian	Code			Colour
Yin and Yang *Black and White*	Ren mai: Controller vessel	CV	▭ ▭		*Black or Blue*
	Du mai: Supervisor vessel	SV	▭▭		*White or Red*
Water *Blue and Black*	Kidney meridian	KD	▭ ▭		*Cyan*
	Bladder meridian	BL	▭▭		*Dark Blue*
Wood *Green and Yellow*	Liver meridian	LV	▭ ▭		*Light Green*
	Gall Bladder meridian	GB	▭▭		*Dark green*
Fire i *Red and Purple*	Heart meridian	HT	▭ ▭		*Deep Pink*
	Small Intestine meridian	SI	▭▭		*Red*
Fire ii *Red and Purple*	Heart Governor meridian	HG	▭ ▭		*Orange*
	Triple Heater meridian	TH	▭▭		*Purple*
Earth *Brown and Yellow*	Spleen meridian	SP	▭ ▭		*Yellow*
	Stomach meridian	ST	▭▭		*Brown*
Metal *White and Gold*	Lung meridian	LU	▭ ▭		*White or Gold*
	Large Intestine meridian	LI	▭▭		*Grey or Silver*

▭   ▭   ▭   Yin meridian

▭▭   Yang meridian

▭●▭   UK Shiatsu Society study point for location and function only

▭◉▭   UK Shiatsu Society study point for location only

ST ▭—○ ST-12   Traditional point on same meridian (Stomach 12 on Stomach meridian)

ST ▭—○ TH-2   Traditional point on other meridian (Triple Heater 2 on Stomach meridian)

▭⊗▭   Traditional extra-ordinary point on meridian

▭⊗▭   Author's extra-ordinary point on meridian (non-traditional)

▭ ▭ ▭ (HT)   Hara (abdomen) or Back diagnostic zone: Lightly colour as related meridian

⬭   Muscle: Leave *shaded*. Tendon: Leave *White*

⬯   Skeletal Bones: Leave *shaded*

▭▭▭
4   3   2   1   0

Oriental anatomical inch ruler: Leave *shaded* or colour *Blue*
Chinese unit = Cun   Japanese unit = Sun
Unit is derived from the width of receiver's thumb at the interphalangeal joint

Chapter 1
ANATOMY
Measurement
Skeleton
Muscles
and
Organs

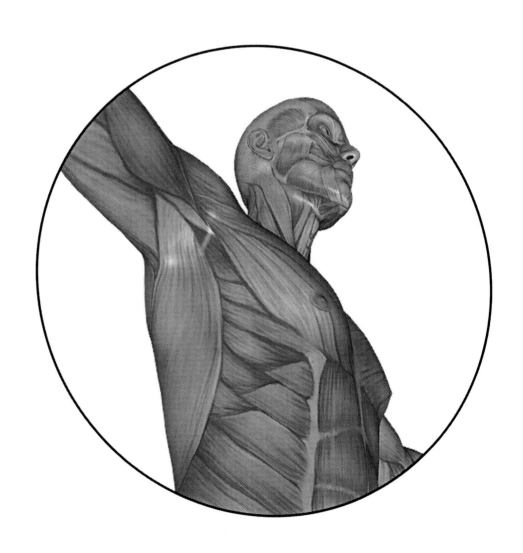

Proportional measurement

The traditional Chinese anatomical inch or cun is employed throughout this book to accurately locate the standard xue or points for treatment and proportionately scale the Human body.

Fundamentally, with regard to the person being treated, one unit or cun is equal to the widest part of their thumb's inter-phalangeal joint.
For greater fluency and scope in practice however, other combinations of the fingers are useful. These location methods and the scales of this system of measurement are annotated and illustrated here and overleaf respectfully.

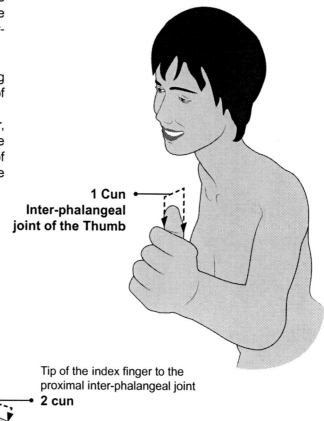

1 Cun
Inter-phalangeal
joint of the Thumb

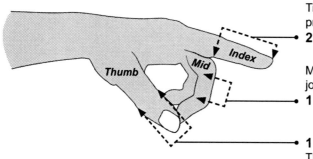

Tip of the index finger to the proximal inter-phalangeal joint
2 cun

Middle finger's inter-phalangeal joint between the end creases
1 cun

1 cun
Thumb's widest part at the inter-phalangeal joint

Middle and index fingers held together

Level with the middle finger's dorsal crease of the proximal inter-phalangeal joint
1.5 cun

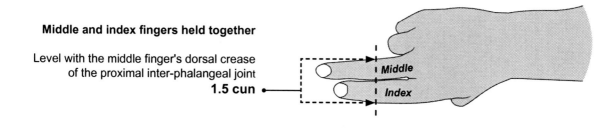

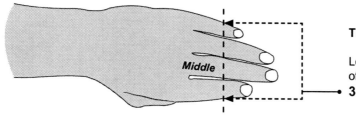

The four fingers held together

Level with the middle finger's dorsal crease of the proximal inter-phalangeal joint
3 cun

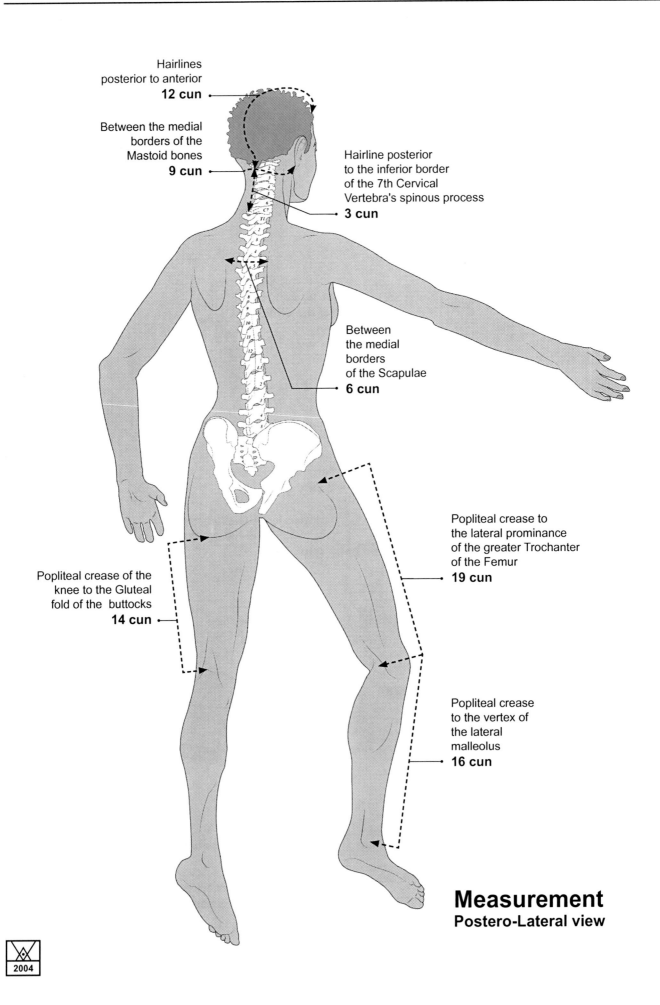

Hairlines
posterior to anterior
12 cun

Between the medial
borders of the
Mastoid bones
9 cun

Hairline posterior
to the inferior border
of the 7th Cervical
Vertebra's spinous process
3 cun

Between
the medial
borders
of the Scapulae
6 cun

Popliteal crease to
the lateral prominance
of the greater Trochanter
of the Femur
19 cun

Popliteal crease of the
knee to the Gluteal
fold of the buttocks
14 cun

Popliteal crease
to the vertex of
the lateral
malleolus
16 cun

Measurement
Postero-Lateral view

2004

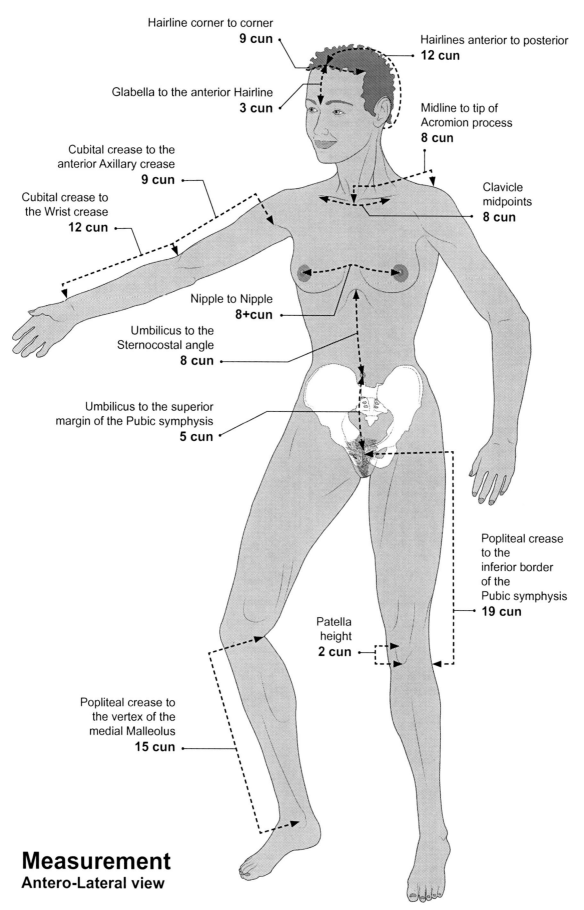

Hairline corner to corner
9 cun

Hairlines anterior to posterior
12 cun

Glabella to the anterior Hairline
3 cun

Midline to tip of
Acromion process
8 cun

Cubital crease to the
anterior Axillary crease
9 cun

Clavicle
midpoints
8 cun

Cubital crease to
the Wrist crease
12 cun

Nipple to Nipple
8+cun

Umbilicus to the
Sternocostal angle
8 cun

Umbilicus to the superior
margin of the Pubic symphysis
5 cun

Popliteal crease
to the
inferior border
of the
Pubic symphysis
19 cun

Patella
height
2 cun

Popliteal crease to
the vertex of the
medial Malleolus
15 cun

Measurement
Antero-Lateral view

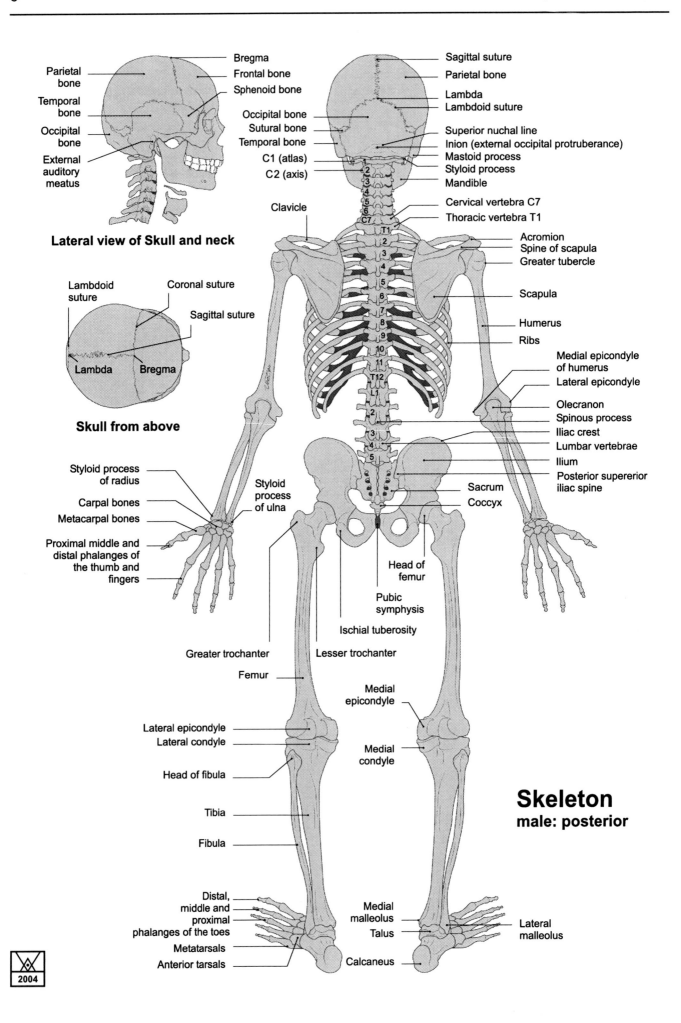

Lateral view of Skull and neck

Skull from above

Skeleton
male: posterior

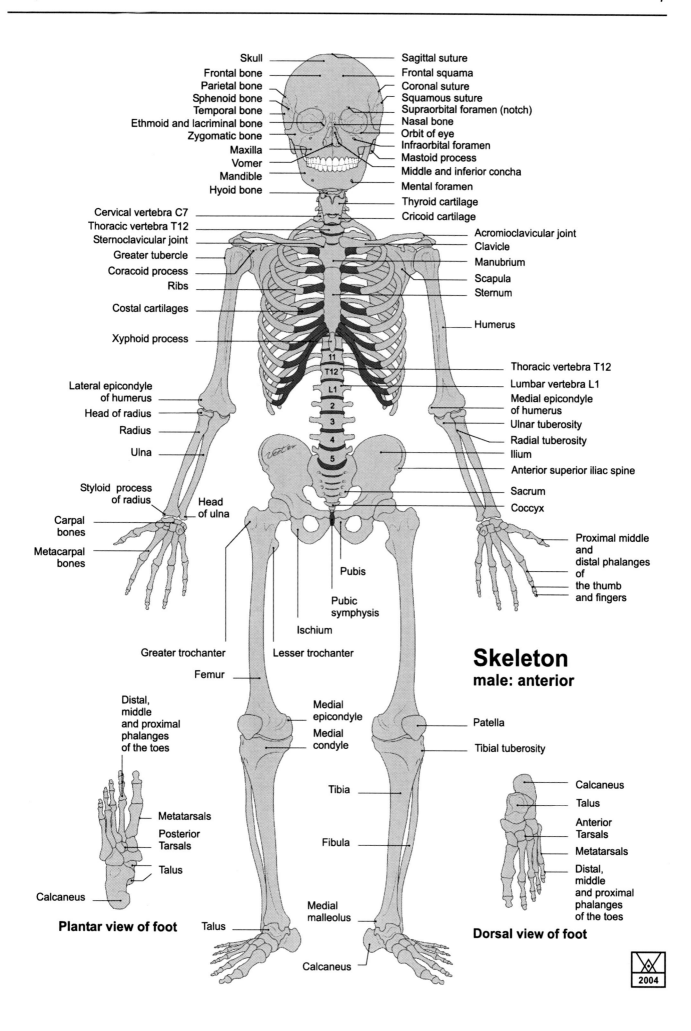

Skull
Frontal bone
Parietal bone
Sphenoid bone
Temporal bone
Ethmoid and lacrimal bone
Zygomatic bone
Maxilla
Vomer
Mandible
Hyoid bone

Sagittal suture
Frontal squama
Coronal suture
Squamous suture
Supraorbital foramen (notch)
Nasal bone
Orbit of eye
Infraorbital foramen
Mastoid process
Middle and inferior concha
Mental foramen
Thyroid cartilage
Cricoid cartilage

Cervical vertebra C7
Thoracic vertebra T12
Sternoclavicular joint
Greater tubercle
Coracoid process
Ribs
Costal cartilages
Xyphoid process

Acromioclavicular joint
Clavicle
Manubrium
Scapula
Sternum

Humerus

11
T12
L1
2
3
4
5

Thoracic vertebra T12
Lumbar vertebra L1
Medial epicondyle of humerus
Ulnar tuberosity
Radial tuberosity
Ilium
Anterior superior iliac spine
Sacrum
Coccyx

Lateral epicondyle of humerus
Head of radius
Radius
Ulna

Styloid process of radius
Carpal bones
Metacarpal bones

Head of ulna

Proximal middle and distal phalanges of the thumb and fingers

Pubis

Pubic symphysis

Ischium

Greater trochanter
Femur

Lesser trochanter

Skeleton
male: anterior

Distal, middle and proximal phalanges of the toes

Medial epicondyle
Medial condyle

Patella

Tibial tuberosity

Tibia

Metatarsals
Posterior Tarsals
Talus

Fibula

Calcaneus

Calcaneus
Talus
Anterior Tarsals
Metatarsals
Distal, middle and proximal phalanges of the toes

Plantar view of foot

Talus

Medial malleolus

Calcaneus

Dorsal view of foot

2004

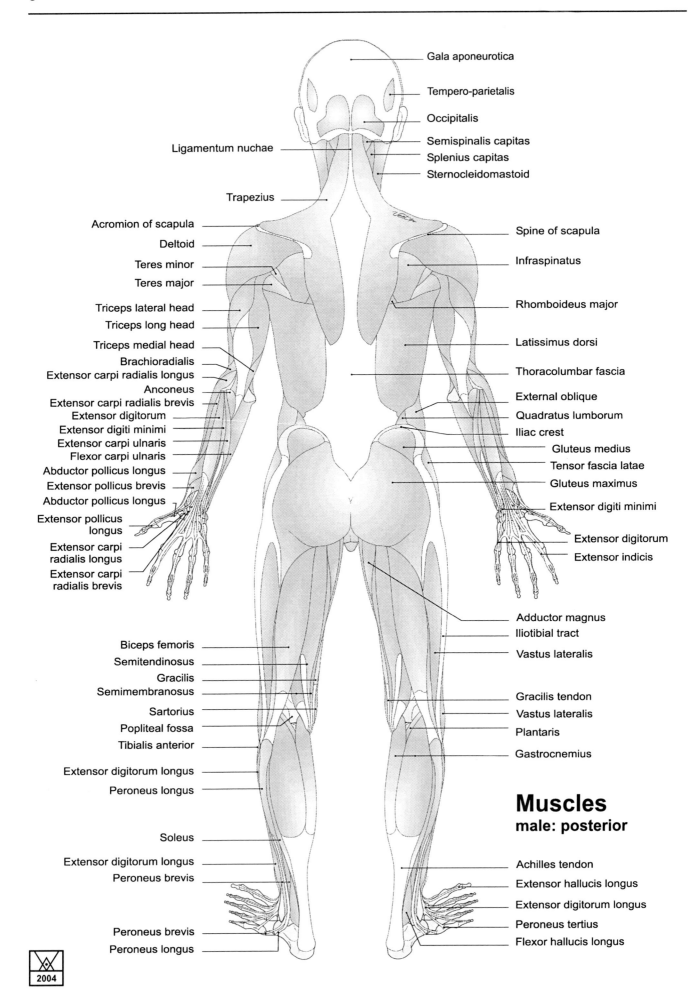

Gala aponeurotica

Tempero-parietalis

Occipitalis

Semispinalis capitas

Splenius capitas

Sternocleidomastoid

Ligamentum nuchae

Trapezius

Acromion of scapula

Deltoid

Teres minor

Teres major

Triceps lateral head

Triceps long head

Triceps medial head

Brachioradialis

Extensor carpi radialis longus

Anconeus

Extensor carpi radialis brevis

Extensor digitorum

Extensor digiti minimi

Extensor carpi ulnaris

Flexor carpi ulnaris

Abductor pollicus longus

Extensor pollicus brevis

Abductor pollicus longus

Extensor pollicus
longus

Extensor carpi
radialis longus

Extensor carpi
radialis brevis

Spine of scapula

Infraspinatus

Rhomboideus major

Latissimus dorsi

Thoracolumbar fascia

External oblique

Quadratus lumborum

Iliac crest

Gluteus medius

Tensor fascia latae

Gluteus maximus

Extensor digiti minimi

Extensor digitorum

Extensor indicis

Biceps femoris

Semitendinosus

Gracilis

Semimembranosus

Sartorius

Popliteal fossa

Tibialis anterior

Extensor digitorum longus

Peroneus longus

Soleus

Extensor digitorum longus

Peroneus brevis

Peroneus brevis

Peroneus longus

Adductor magnus

Iliotibial tract

Vastus lateralis

Gracilis tendon

Vastus lateralis

Plantaris

Gastrocnemius

Muscles
male: posterior

Achilles tendon

Extensor hallucis longus

Extensor digitorum longus

Peroneus tertius

Flexor hallucis longus

2004

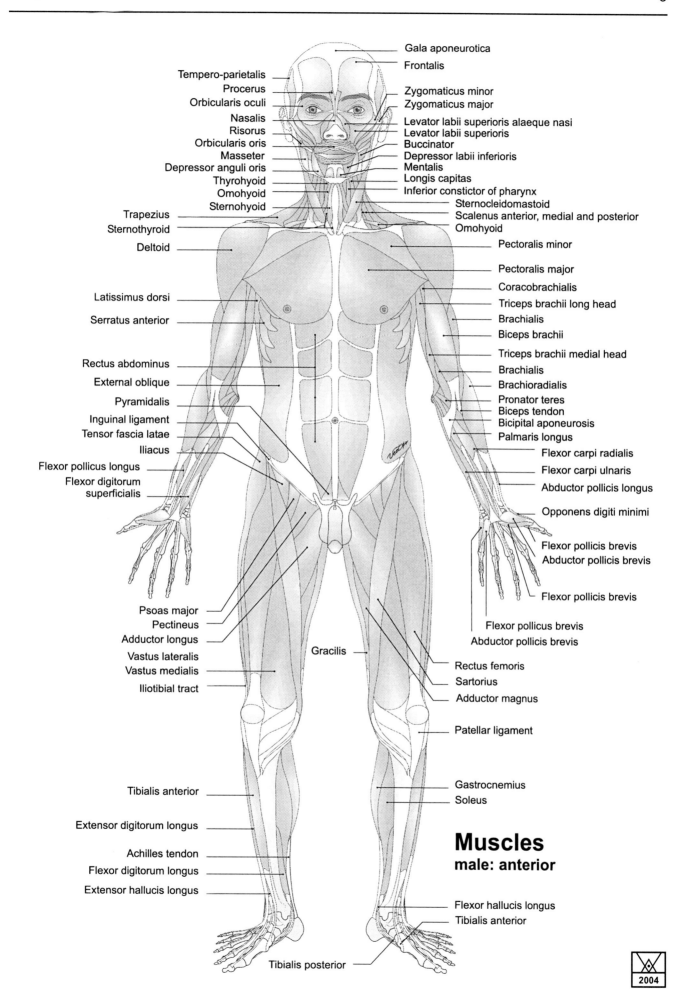

Gala aponeurotica
Frontalis
Tempero-parietalis
Procerus
Orbicularis oculi
Zygomaticus minor
Zygomaticus major
Nasalis
Levator labii superioris alaeque nasi
Risorus
Levator labii superioris
Orbicularis oris
Buccinator
Masseter
Depressor labii inferioris
Depressor anguli oris
Mentalis
Thyrohyoid
Longis capitas
Omohyoid
Inferior constictor of pharynx
Sternohyoid
Sternocleidomastoid
Trapezius
Scalenus anterior, medial and posterior
Sternothyroid
Omohyoid
Deltoid
Pectoralis minor
Pectoralis major
Coracobrachialis
Latissimus dorsi
Triceps brachii long head
Serratus anterior
Brachialis
Biceps brachii
Triceps brachii medial head
Rectus abdominus
Brachialis
External oblique
Brachioradialis
Pyramidalis
Pronator teres
Inguinal ligament
Biceps tendon
Tensor fascia latae
Bicipital aponeurosis
Iliacus
Palmaris longus
Flexor pollicus longus
Flexor carpi radialis
Flexor digitorum
Flexor carpi ulnaris
superficialis
Abductor pollicis longus
Opponens digiti minimi
Flexor pollicis brevis
Abductor pollicis brevis
Flexor pollicis brevis
Psoas major
Flexor pollicus brevis
Pectineus
Abductor pollicis brevis
Adductor longus
Vastus lateralis
Gracilis
Vastus medialis
Rectus femoris
Iliotibial tract
Sartorius
Adductor magnus
Patellar ligament
Gastrocnemius
Tibialis anterior
Soleus
Extensor digitorum longus
Achilles tendon
Flexor digitorum longus
Extensor hallucis longus

Muscles
male: anterior

Flexor hallucis longus
Tibialis anterior
Tibialis posterior

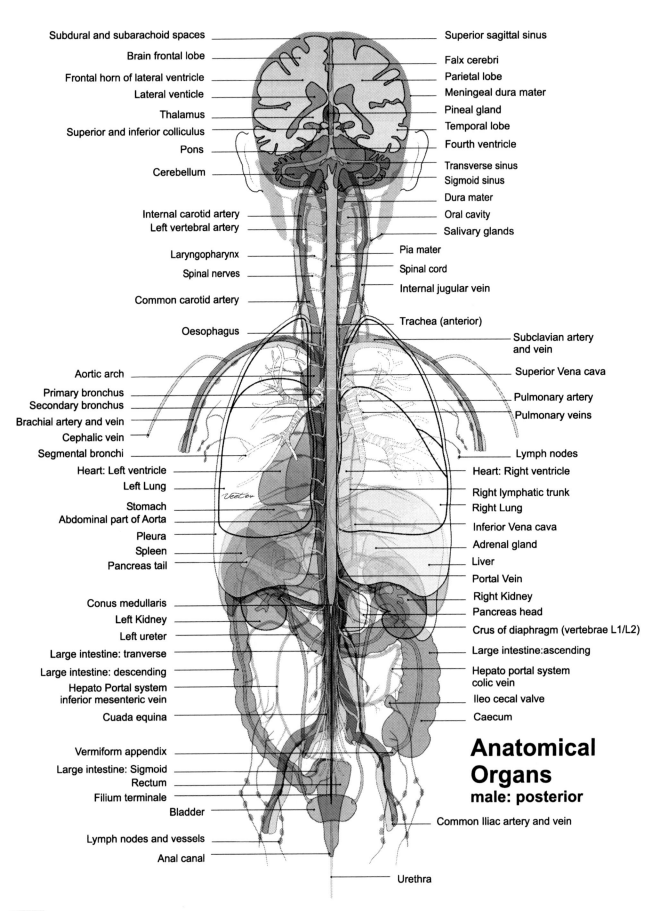

Subdural and subarachoid spaces

Brain frontal lobe

Frontal horn of lateral ventricle

Lateral venticle

Thalamus

Superior and inferior colliculus

Pons

Cerebellum

Internal carotid artery

Left vertebral artery

Laryngopharynx

Spinal nerves

Common carotid artery

Oesophagus

Aortic arch

Primary bronchus

Secondary bronchus

Brachial artery and vein

Cephalic vein

Segmental bronchi

Heart: Left ventricle

Left Lung

Stomach

Abdominal part of Aorta

Pleura

Spleen

Pancreas tail

Conus medullaris

Left Kidney

Left ureter

Large intestine: tranverse

Large intestine: descending

Hepato Portal system
inferior mesenteric vein

Cuada equina

Vermiform appendix

Large intestine: Sigmoid

Rectum

Filium terminale

Bladder

Lymph nodes and vessels

Anal canal

Superior sagittal sinus

Falx cerebri

Parietal lobe

Meningeal dura mater

Pineal gland

Temporal lobe

Fourth ventricle

Transverse sinus

Sigmoid sinus

Dura mater

Oral cavity

Salivary glands

Pia mater

Spinal cord

Internal jugular vein

Trachea (anterior)

Subclavian artery
and vein

Superior Vena cava

Pulmonary artery

Pulmonary veins

Lymph nodes

Heart: Right ventricle

Right lymphatic trunk

Right Lung

Inferior Vena cava

Adrenal gland

Liver

Portal Vein

Right Kidney

Pancreas head

Crus of diaphragm (vertebrae L1/L2)

Large intestine:ascending

Hepato portal system
colic vein

Ileo cecal valve

Caecum

Anatomical
Organs
male: posterior

Common Iliac artery and vein

Urethra

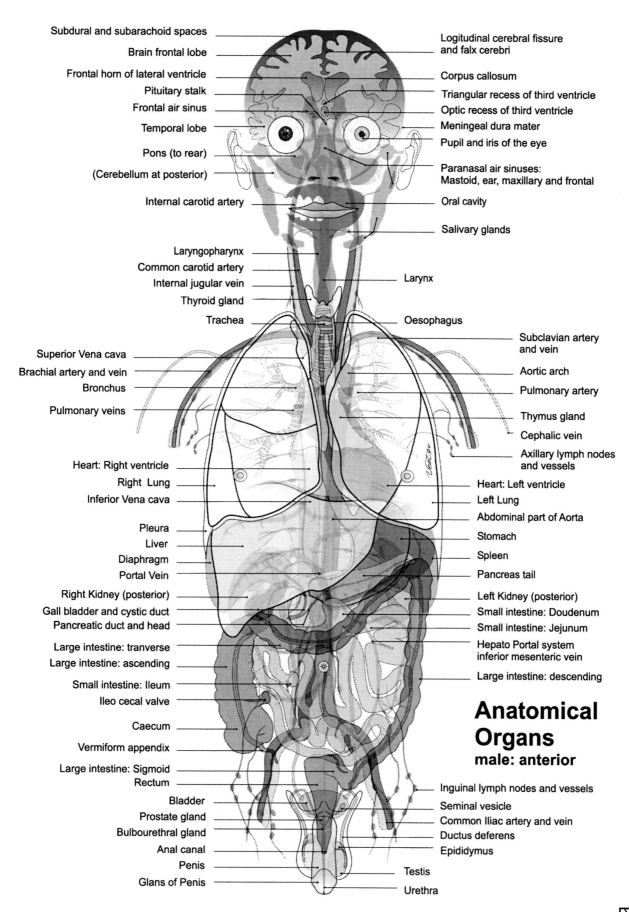

Subdural and subarachoid spaces

Brain frontal lobe

Frontal horn of lateral ventricle

Pituitary stalk

Frontal air sinus

Temporal lobe

Pons (to rear)

(Cerebellum at posterior)

Internal carotid artery

Logitudinal cerebral fissure and falx cerebri

Corpus callosum

Triangular recess of third ventricle

Optic recess of third ventricle

Meningeal dura mater

Pupil and iris of the eye

Paranasal air sinuses:
Mastoid, ear, maxillary and frontal

Oral cavity

Salivary glands

Laryngopharynx

Common carotid artery

Internal jugular vein

Thyroid gland

Trachea

Larynx

Oesophagus

Superior Vena cava

Brachial artery and vein

Bronchus

Pulmonary veins

Subclavian artery and vein

Aortic arch

Pulmonary artery

Thymus gland

Cephalic vein

Axillary lymph nodes and vessels

Heart: Right ventricle

Right Lung

Inferior Vena cava

Pleura

Liver

Diaphragm

Portal Vein

Right Kidney (posterior)

Gall bladder and cystic duct

Pancreatic duct and head

Large intestine: tranverse

Large intestine: ascending

Small intestine: Ileum

Ileo cecal valve

Caecum

Vermiform appendix

Large intestine: Sigmoid

Rectum

Bladder

Prostate gland

Bulbourethral gland

Anal canal

Penis

Glans of Penis

Heart: Left ventricle

Left Lung

Abdominal part of Aorta

Stomach

Spleen

Pancreas tail

Left Kidney (posterior)

Small intestine: Doudenum

Small intestine: Jejunum

Hepato Portal system inferior mesenteric vein

Large intestine: descending

Anatomical Organs
male: anterior

Inguinal lymph nodes and vessels

Seminal vesicle

Common Iliac artery and vein

Ductus deferens

Epididymus

Testis

Urethra

2004

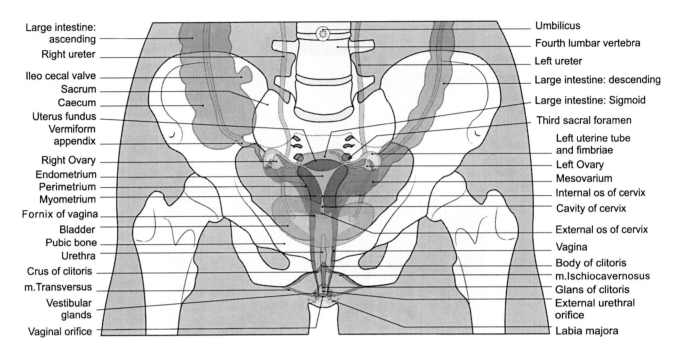

Large intestine: ascending
Right ureter
Ileo cecal valve
Sacrum
Caecum
Uterus fundus
Vermiform appendix
Right Ovary
Endometrium
Perimetrium
Myometrium
Fornix of vagina
Bladder
Pubic bone
Urethra
Crus of clitoris
m.Transversus
Vestibular glands
Vaginal orifice

Umbilicus
Fourth lumbar vertebra
Left ureter
Large intestine: descending
Large intestine: Sigmoid
Third sacral foramen
Left uterine tube and fimbriae
Left Ovary
Mesovarium
Internal os of cervix
Cavity of cervix
External os of cervix
Vagina
Body of clitoris
m.Ischiocavernosus
Glans of clitoris
External urethral orifice
Labia majora

Pelvic Anatomy
female organs: anterior view

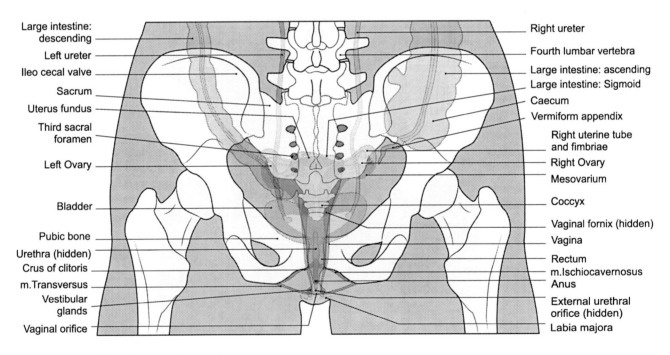

Large intestine: descending
Left ureter
Ileo cecal valve
Sacrum
Uterus fundus
Third sacral foramen
Left Ovary
Bladder
Pubic bone
Urethra (hidden)
Crus of clitoris
m.Transversus
Vestibular glands
Vaginal orifice

Right ureter
Fourth lumbar vertebra
Large intestine: ascending
Large intestine: Sigmoid
Caecum
Vermiform appendix
Right uterine tube and fimbriae
Right Ovary
Mesovarium
Coccyx
Vaginal fornix (hidden)
Vagina
Rectum
m.Ischiocavernosus
Anus
External urethral orifice (hidden)
Labia majora

Pelvic Anatomy
female organs: posterior view

Chapter 2
DIAGNOSTICS

Classical Chinese medicine
and
Zen Shiatsu systems

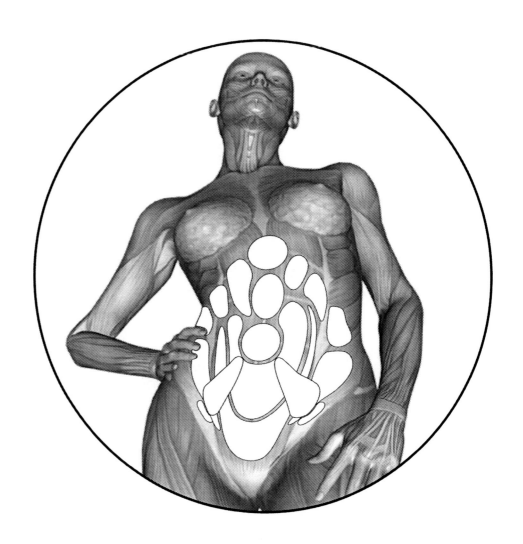

Table 2.1 The basic Yin and Yang correspondences

Modes	YANG 陽	YIN 陰
ENVIRONMENTAL	Heaven Round Sun Time Light Midday, Day Above Hot Fire East, South Spring, Summer	Earth Flat Moon Space Darkness Midnight, Night Below Cold Water West, North Autumn, Winter
MOVEMENT	Creative Activity Ascending Expanding Evaporating Visible Repletion Birth, Child-Adulthood, Gestation	Receptive Stillness Descending Contracting Condensing Hidden Depletion Mid-Old Age, Death, Conception
BODY	Male External, Back and Upper body Left Side of body Stomach, Gall Bladder, Large Intestine, Small Intestine, Bladder Brain and Cranium Cervical and Thoracic spine Shoulder, Arms and Hands	Female Internal, Front and Lower body Right Side of body Lungs, Heart, Liver, Spleen, Kidneys Abdomen, and Pelvis Sacral and Lumbar spine Hips, Legs and Feet
DIAGNOSTICS	Acute conditions Excess Flushed complexion Feel Hot and/or Dry Agitated Firm and/or Light Body Loud Voice Talkative Red and Dry Tongue Involves Nerves Immunity and Thermo-dynamics Excretion of Nutrient waste Transportation of Nutrients	Chronic conditions Deficiency Pale complexion Feel Cold and/or Damp Lethargic Soft and/or Heavy Body Weak Voice Silent Pale and Wet Tongue Involves Blood Hormones and Fluids Intake of Nutrients Transformation of Nutrients

Fig. 2.1 Classical facial diagnostic zones and indications

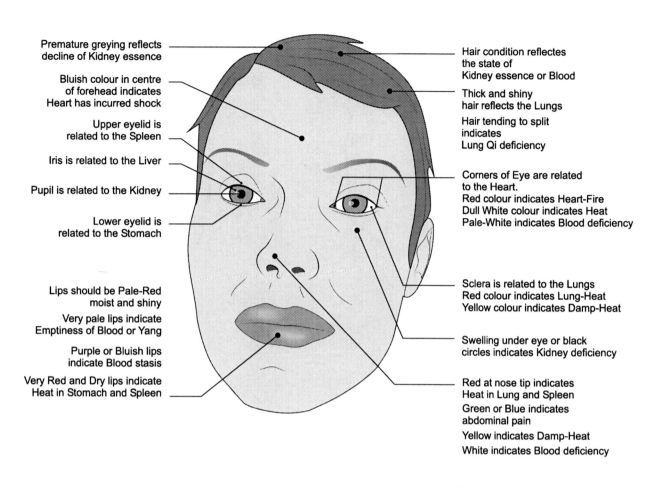

Premature greying reflects decline of Kidney essence

Bluish colour in centre of forehead indicates Heart has incurred shock

Upper eyelid is related to the Spleen

Iris is related to the Liver

Pupil is related to the Kidney

Lower eyelid is related to the Stomach

Lips should be Pale-Red moist and shiny

Very pale lips indicate Emptiness of Blood or Yang

Purple or Bluish lips indicate Blood stasis

Very Red and Dry lips indicate Heat in Stomach and Spleen

Hair condition reflects the state of Kidney essence or Blood

Thick and shiny hair reflects the Lungs

Hair tending to split indicates Lung Qi deficiency

Corners of Eye are related to the Heart.
Red colour indicates Heart-Fire
Dull White colour indicates Heat
Pale-White indicates Blood deficiency

Sclera is related to the Lungs
Red colour indicates Lung-Heat
Yellow colour indicates Damp-Heat

Swelling under eye or black circles indicates Kidney deficiency

Red at nose tip indicates Heat in Lung and Spleen
Green or Blue indicates abdominal pain
Yellow indicates Damp-Heat
White indicates Blood deficiency

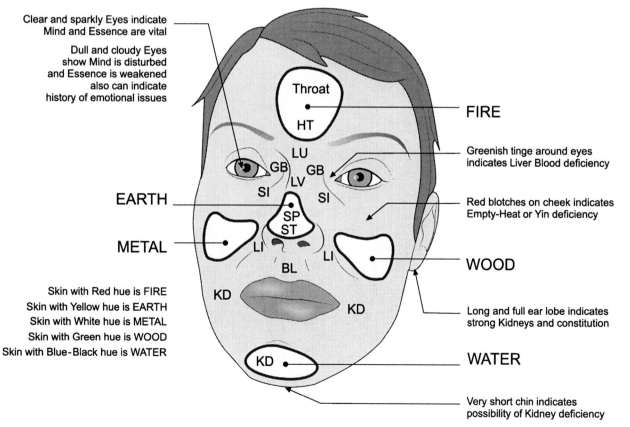

Clear and sparkly Eyes indicate Mind and Essence are vital

Dull and cloudy Eyes show Mind is disturbed and Essence is weakened also can indicate history of emotional issues

EARTH

METAL

Skin with Red hue is FIRE
Skin with Yellow hue is EARTH
Skin with White hue is METAL
Skin with Green hue is WOOD
Skin with Blue-Black hue is WATER

Throat
HT
LU
GB GB
LV
SI   SI
SP
ST
LI   LI
BL
KD   KD
KD

FIRE

Greenish tinge around eyes indicates Liver Blood deficiency

Red blotches on cheek indicates Empty-Heat or Yin deficiency

WOOD

Long and full ear lobe indicates strong Kidneys and constitution

WATER

Very short chin indicates possibility of Kidney deficiency

Fig. 2.2 Classical tongue diagnostic zones and indications

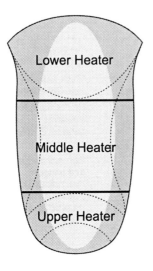 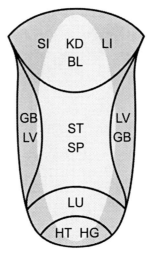 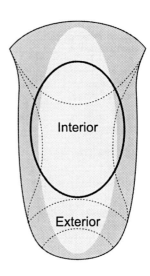

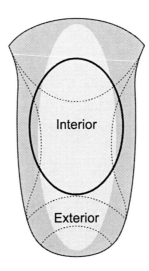

Interior conditions
Reflected on tongue body
via colour and shape

Interior/Exterior conditions
White coating to one side or front
Black or grey coating to back

Exterior conditions
Wind-Cold, front has white coating
Wind-Heat, front has yellow coating
Thicker coating indicates stregth of pathogen

Excess conditions
Stiff, swollen tongue body thick coating
Cold has pale body, slippery white coating
Heat has red body, thick yellow coating
Purple body is stasis of blood
Phlegm is thick, greasy and slippery coating

Deficiency conditions
Pale tongue body in Yang / Blood deficiency
Red tongue body in Yin deficiency
Tongue body shape is thin/flaccid, no coating

Hot conditions
Red tongue body and yellow coating

Cold conditions
Pale tongue body and white coating

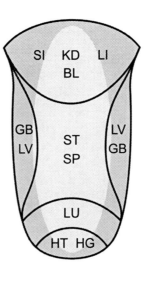

Yin deficiency
KD: red tongue body, cracks, dry, no coating
ST: centre has dry wide crack, no coating
LU: red tongue body, front cracks , no coating
HT: red tongue body and tip redder, no coating

Yang deficiency
KD: pale tongue body, swollen, white coating
SP: pale tongue body, wet, no coating
HT: pale tongue body,
severe if blue-purple color

Qi deficiency
ST: absence of coating at tongue centre
SP: teeth marks on tongue inc sides
LU: tongue anterior swollen and flaccid
HT: pale tongue body

Blood deficiency
LV: pale tongue body with paler sides
SP: pale tongue body and a little dry
HT: pale tongue body with paler tip

Fig. 2.3 Classical pulse positions and depths

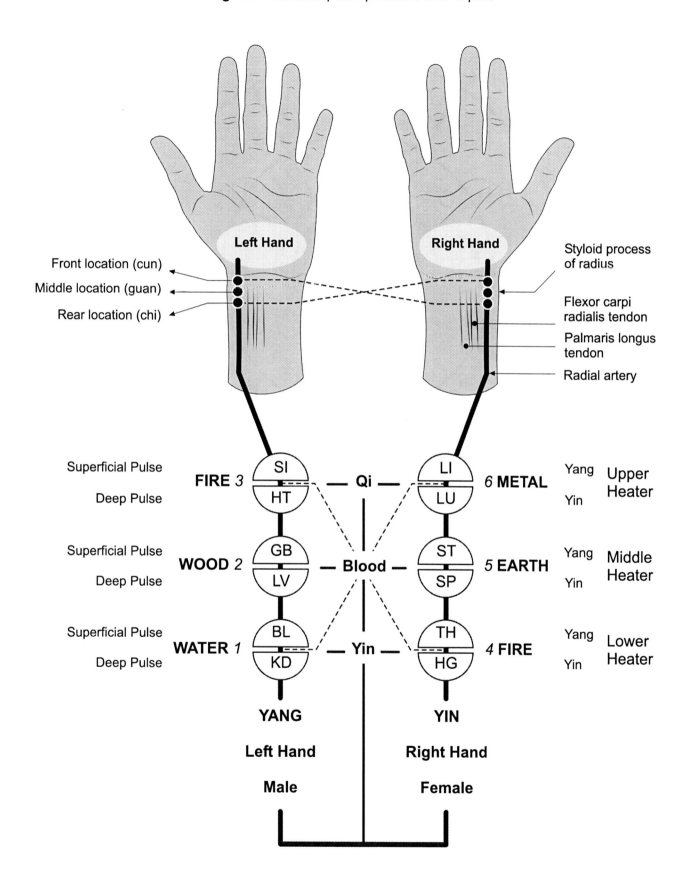

Fig. 2.4 Chinese clock indicating peak flow of Qi through channels and vessels

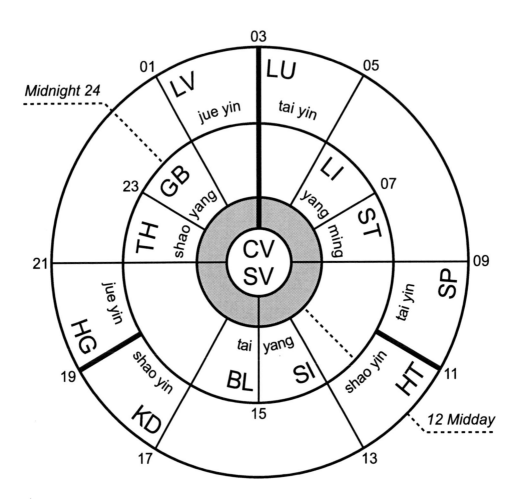

Table 2.2 Classification and routes of Qi flow per Zangfu and vessels

Yin-Yang identity	Channel or vessel route	Zangfu and vessels
Tai yin	Chest to Hand	Lung
Yang ming	Hand to Face	Large Intestine
Yang ming	Face to Foot	Stomach
Tai yin	Foot to Chest	Spleen
Shao yin	Chest to Hand	Heart
Tai yang	Hand to Face	Small Intestine
Tai yang	Face to Foot	Bladder
Shao yin	Foot to Chest	Kidney
Jue yin	Chest to Hand	Heart Governor
Shao yang	Hand to Face	Triple Heater
Shao yang	Face to Foot	Gall Bladder
Jue yin	Foot to Chest	Liver
Yang	Face, spine to Perineum	Supervisor vessel
Yin	Perineum to Face	Controller vessel

Fig. 2.5 Distribution of the vital substances and source or Yuan Qi

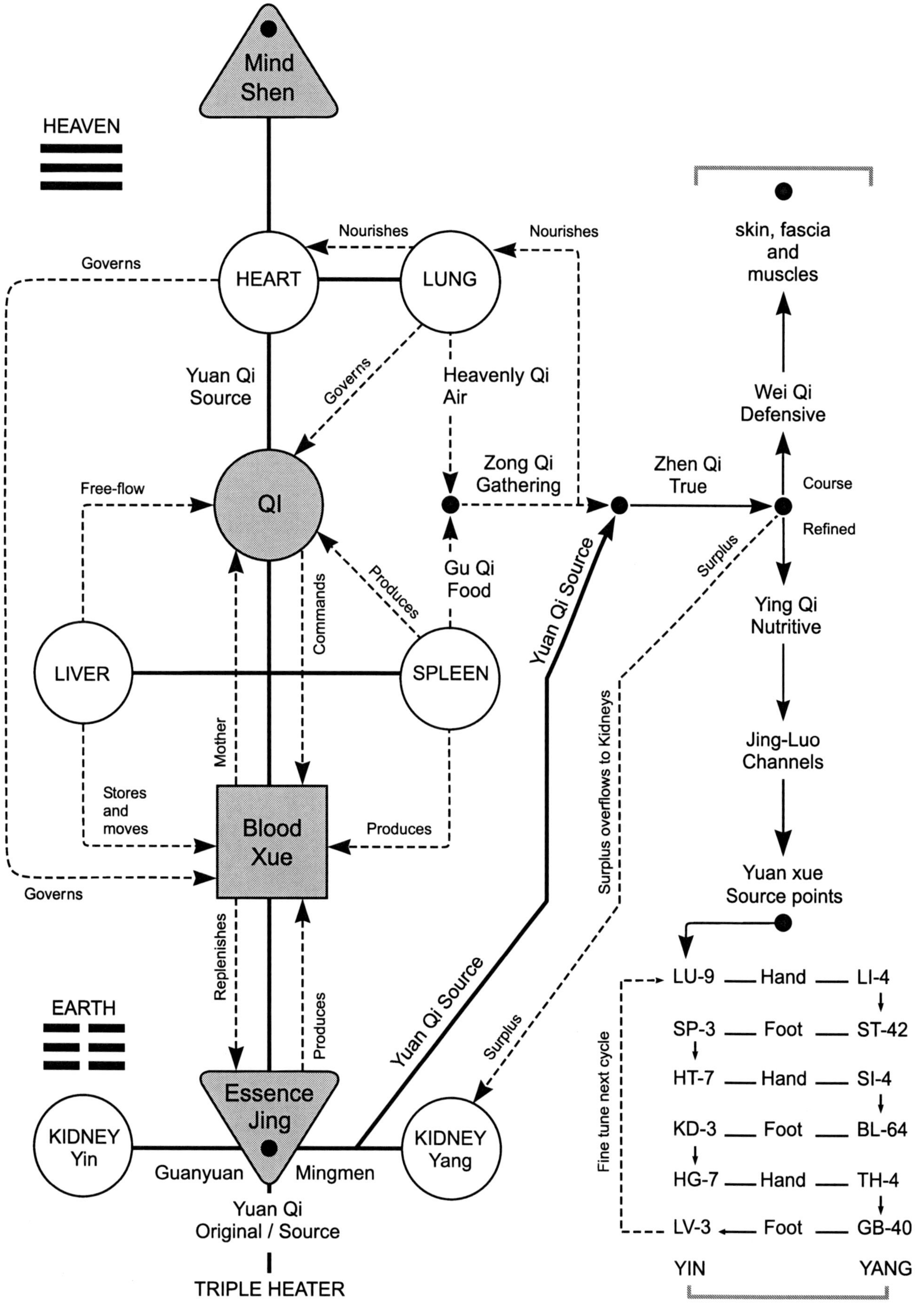

Fig. 2.6 Shu xue: Transporting points

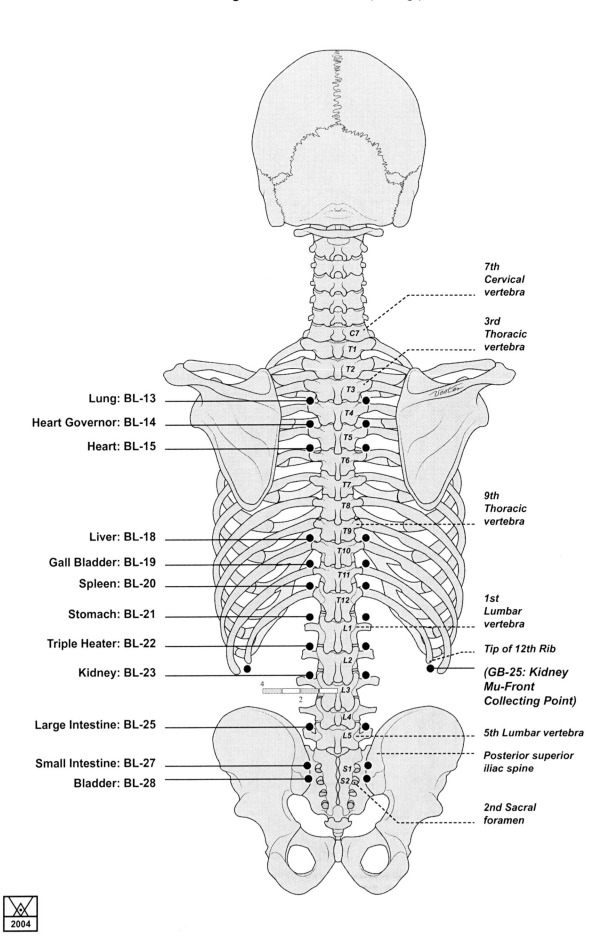

Fig. 2.7 Mu xue: Collecting points

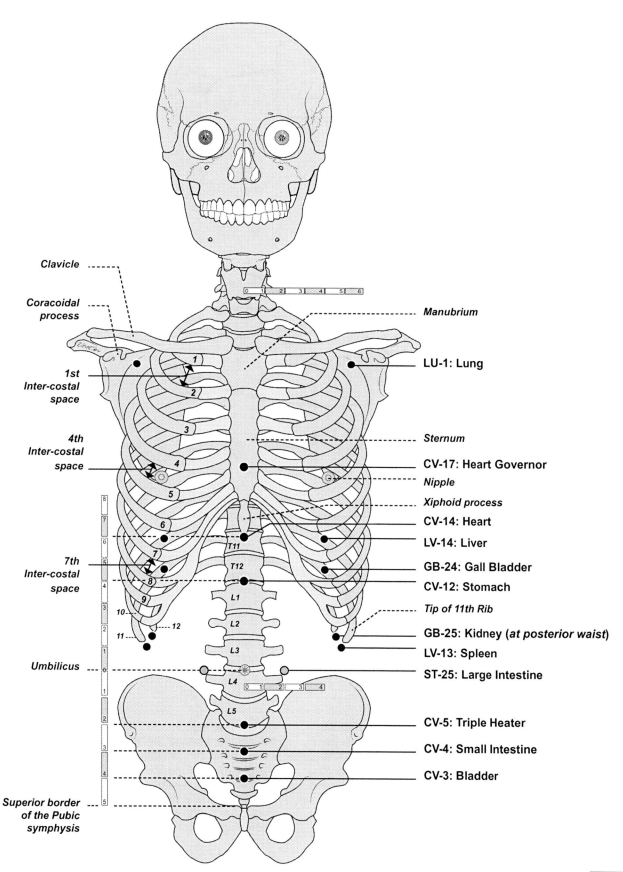

Fig. 2.8 Yin-Yang to Five elements: Cosmological creation sequence

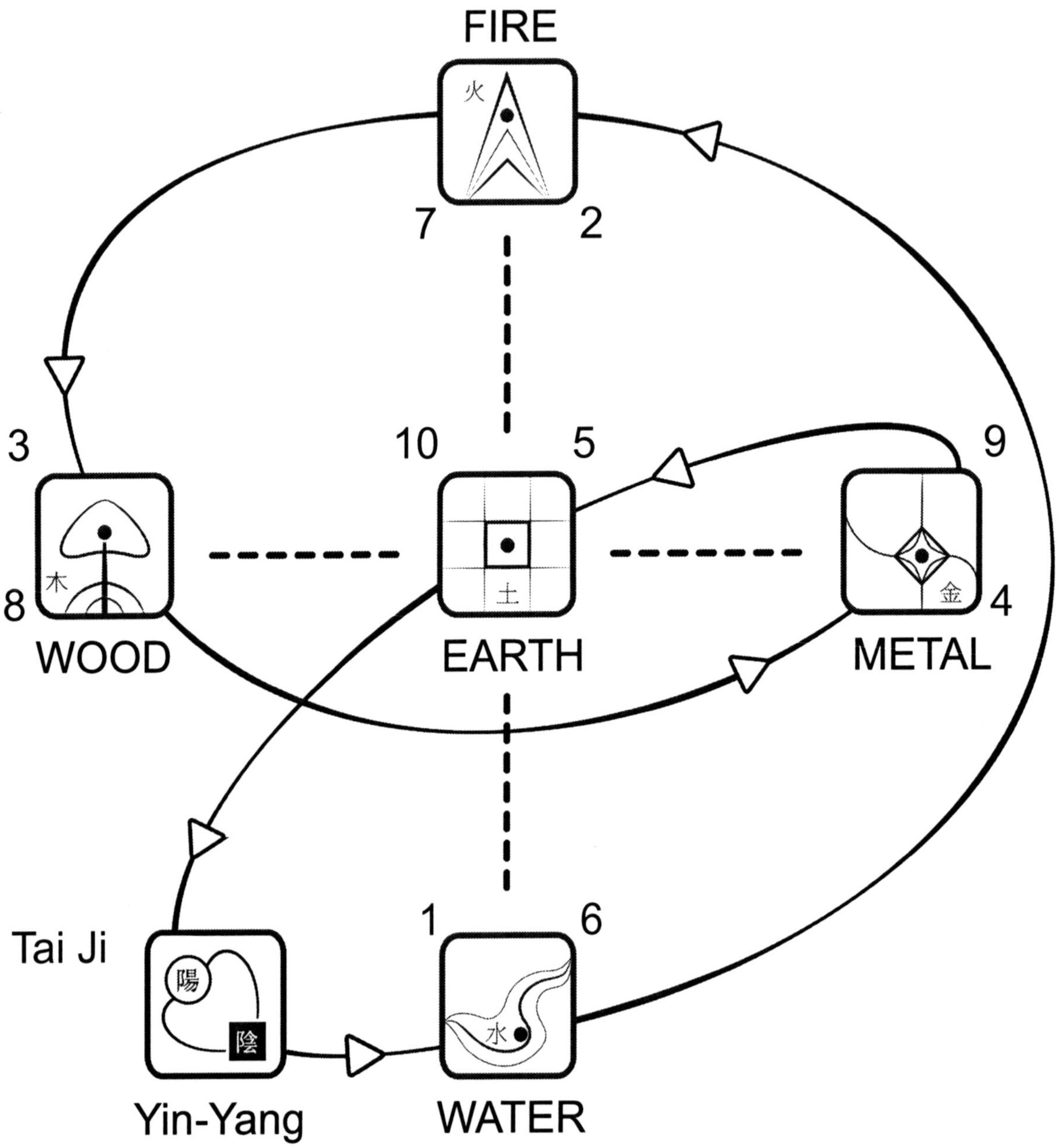

FIRE

7   2

3

10   5   9

8 WOOD   EARTH   METAL 4

Tai Ji

1   6

Yin-Yang   WATER

"The concept of the Five elements was popular during the the period of Warring States (475-221 B.C). At the very beginning, its principle was simple and plain. Before the Han dynasty (206 B.C. – A.D. 220) the I Ching had no connection with the Five elements. It was in the Han dynasty that scholars of the Symbol and Number School began to integrate the Eight Primary Gua (hexagrams) with yin and yang, five elements, eight directions, four seasons, the days and the months, and the parts of the human body, and applied them to medicine, the calendar, astrology, and astronomy."

"Because Water is cold and runs downward, the Water element was placed on the bottom of the picture which, to the ancient Chinese, represented the cold north. Because heat and fire rise, the Fire element was placed on the top of the picture, representing the warm south. Wood flourishes in the east, and thus the Wood element was placed on the left side of the picture representing the east. Because metal was abundant in the western part of China, the Metal element was placed on the right side of the picture, representing the west. Because the energy represented by the Earth element is able to harmonize all other elements, it was placed in the centre."

Master Alfred Huang,
'The Numerology of the I Ching',
p25-26, Inner Traditions International, 2000

Table 2.3 The basic Five element correspondences

Elements / Modes	WATER 水	WOOD 木	FIRE 火	EARTH 土	METAL 金
Spiritual Faculty	Zhi Will	Hun Ethereal soul	Shen Spirit-Mind	Yi Thought	Po Corporeal soul
Yin-Yang	Utmost Yin	Lesser Yang	Utmost Yang	Centre	Lesser Yin
Cycle	Storage	Birth	Growth	Maturity	Harvest
Season	Winter	Spring	Summer	Links seasons	Autumn
Climate	Cold	Wind	Hot	Damp, Humid	Dry
Direction	North	East	South	Centre	West
Colour	Black	Green	Red	Yellow	White
Part of Day	Night	Morning	Midday	Afternoon	Evening
Organ Yin	Kidneys	Liver	Heart	Spleen	Lung
Organ Yang	Bladder	Gall Bladder	Small Intestine	Stomach	Large Intestine
Tissue	Marrow, Bones	Tendons, Ligaments	Blood vessels	Muscle, Flesh	Skin
Odour	Putrid	Rancid	Burning	Fragrant	Rotten
Sense Organ	Ears	Eyes	Tongue	Mouth	Nose
Emotion	Fear, Courage	Anger, Humour	Joy, Hysteria	Empathy, Contemplation	Grief, Positivity
Sound, Voice	Groaning, Humming	Shouting, Clipped	Laughing, Talkative	Singing, Lilting	Weeping, Wailing
Animal	Pig, Fish	Chicken	Sheep, Lamb	Ox, Cow	Horse
Taste	Salty	Sour	Bitter, Hot	Sweet	Spicy
Grain	Beans	Wheat, Barley	Corn	Millet	Rice
Vegetable	Root Plants	Upward growing	Enlarged and Leafy	Round and Sweet	Small and Contracted

Fig. 2.9 The Five elements: Basic sequences

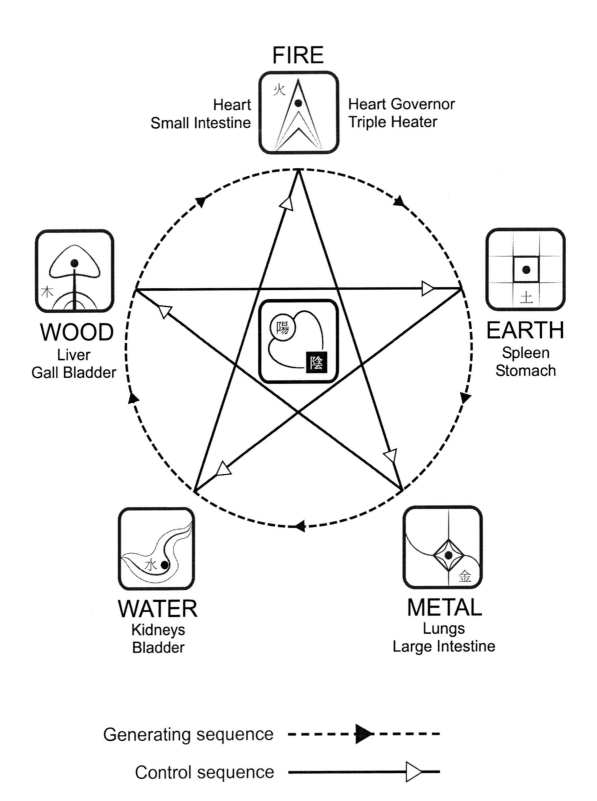

Generating sequence - - - - - ▶ - - - - -

Control sequence ⎯⎯⎯⎯▷

Fig. 2.10 Classification and locale of Five element shu, yuan and luo points

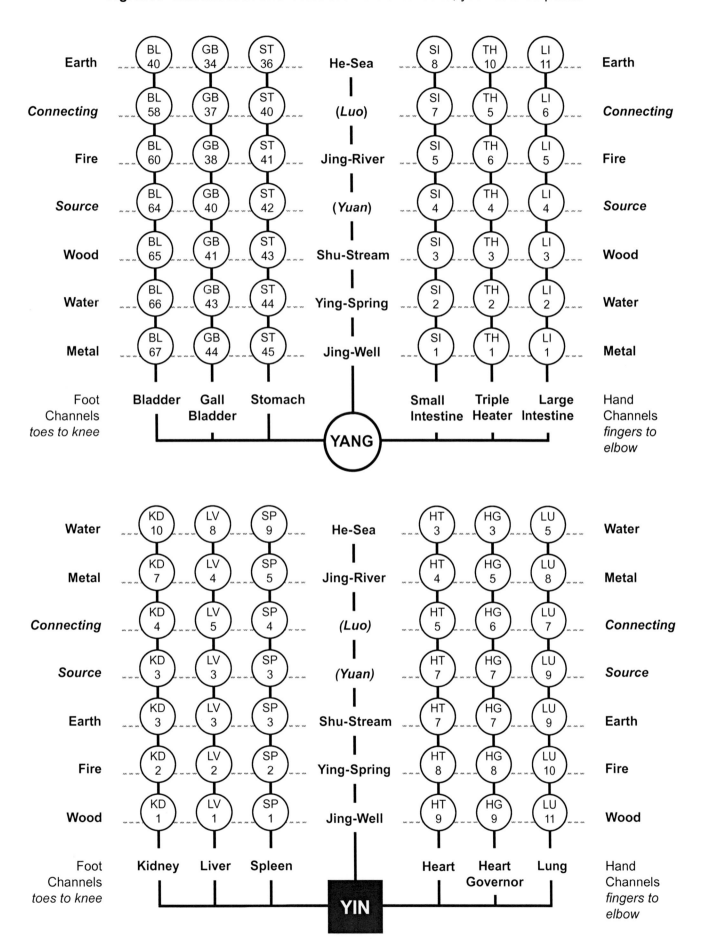

Fig. 2.11 Five element points data and sequence chart

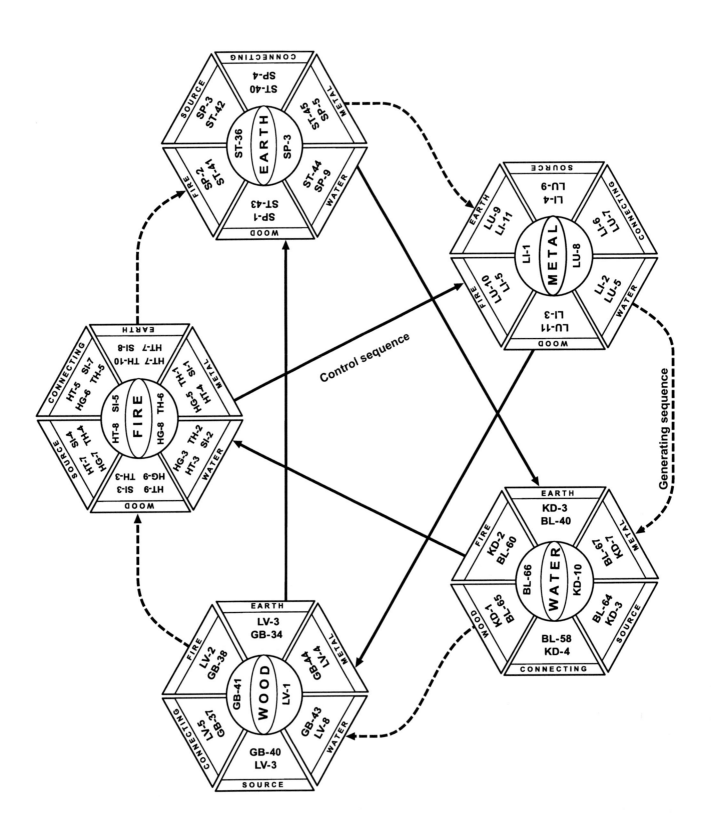

Fig. 2.12 Five element Hara diagnostic zones. Three Heaters and influential points

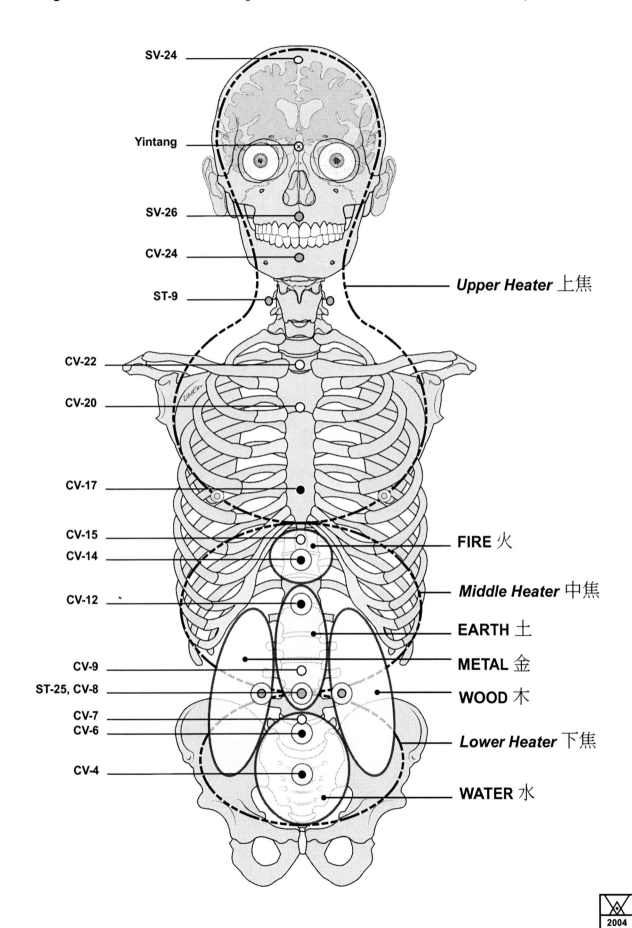

SV-24

Yintang

SV-26

CV-24

ST-9

CV-22

CV-20

CV-17

CV-15
CV-14

CV-12

CV-9

ST-25, CV-8

CV-7
CV-6

CV-4

Upper Heater 上焦

FIRE 火

Middle Heater 中焦

EARTH 土

METAL 金

WOOD 木

Lower Heater 下焦

WATER 水

2004

Fig. 2.13 Zen Shiatsu: Standard Back diagnostic zones

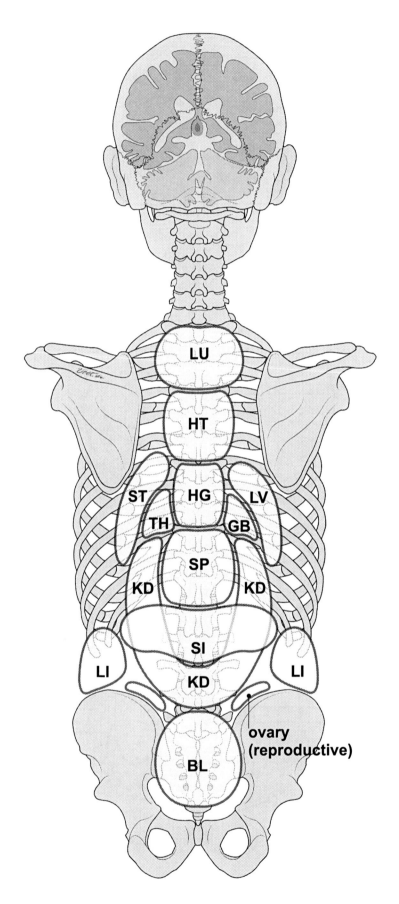

Fig. 2.14 Zen Shiatsu: Standard Hara diagnostic zones

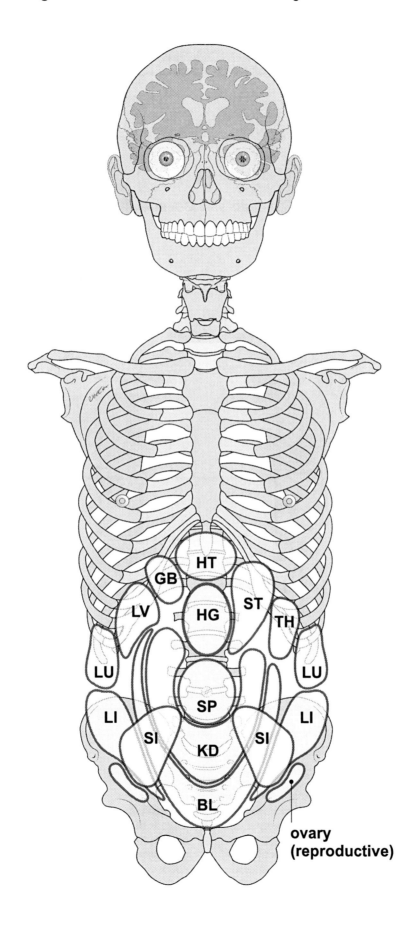

Fig. 2.15 Zen Shiatsu: The primary germ layers and meridian functions (after Masunaga)

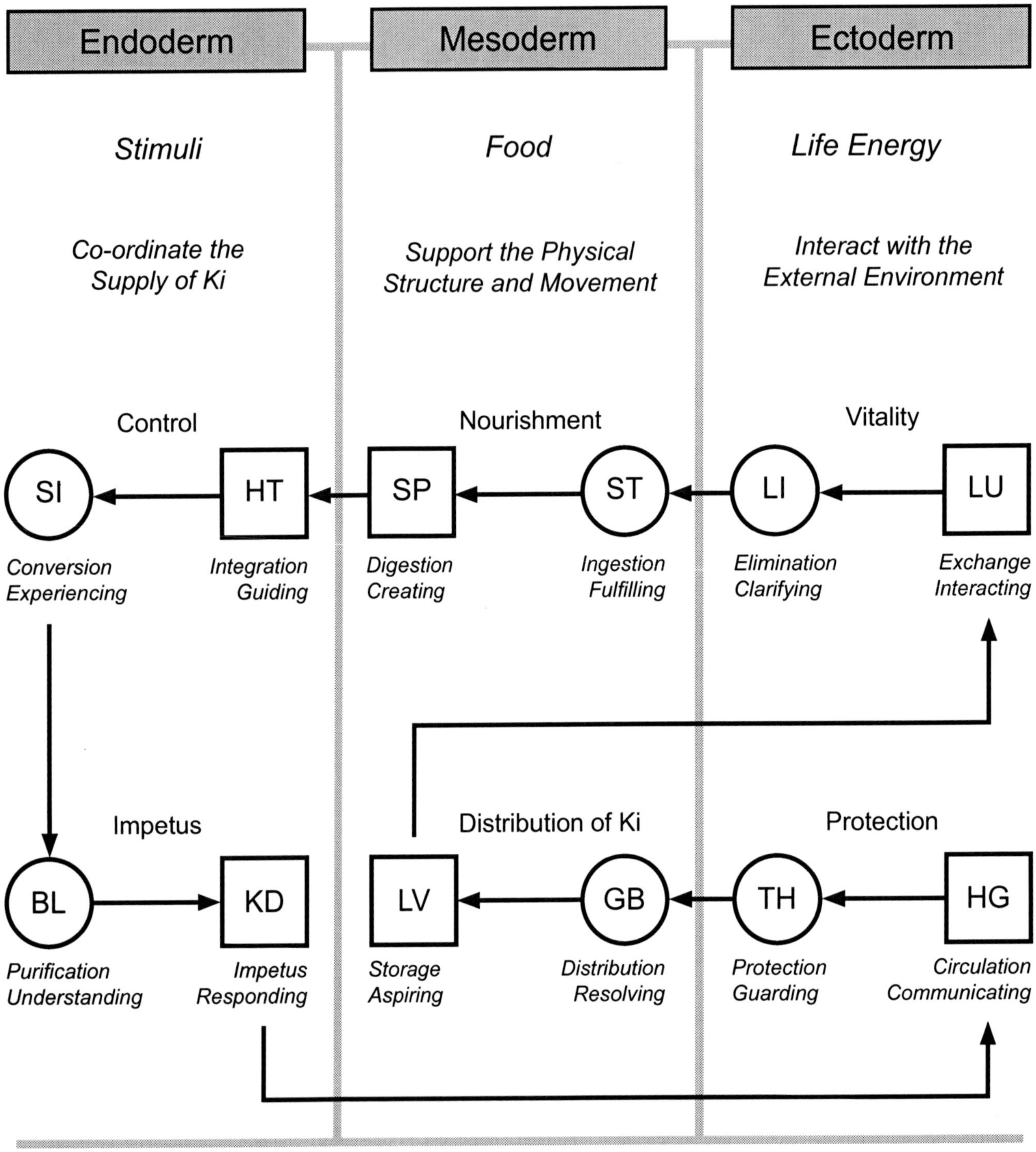

Endoderm	Mesoderm	Ectoderm
Stimuli	*Food*	*Life Energy*
Co-ordinate the Supply of Ki	*Support the Physical Structure and Movement*	*Interact with the External Environment*

Control   Nourishment   Vitality

SI ← HT ← SP ← ST ← LI ← LU

| *Conversion Experiencing* | *Integration Guiding* | *Digestion Creating* | *Ingestion Fulfilling* | *Elimination Clarifying* | *Exchange Interacting* |

Impetus   Distribution of Ki   Protection

BL → KD   LV ← GB ← TH ← HG

| *Purification Understanding* | *Impetus Responding* | *Storage Aspiring* | *Distribution Resolving* | *Protection Guarding* | *Circulation Communicating* |

" In the early stages of embryonic development in higher animals, the mass of stem cells curl up and form a pocket (to contain a small portion of the outside) and the result is the endoderm (which later becomes the internal organs). The part of the embryo which remains directly exposed to the external environment forms the ectoderm (later to become the skin), which serves to provide information about the environment. The mesoderm consists of the inner and outer layers and provides structural support (later becoming the muscles and skeleton). These three layers are just structural specializations of three basic modes of functions which exist in the most primitive single-celled organisms. These three modes of function are represented by the ectoderm, mesoderm, and endoderm and are thus fundamental to all living things."
Shizuto Masunaga,
'Zen Imagery Exercises',
p59-60, Japan Publications, 1987

Fig. 2.16 Zen Shiatsu: Masunagas life cycle of the meridians

VITALITY
Primal life-single cell.
forms an identity.
Skin forms sense of self boundary.
Permeable border for the exchange
of materials.

Exchange and Elimination
**Lung and
Large Intestine**

DISTRIBUTION
How to employ stock of Ki,
nutrients, ideas or emotions.
Take stock of reserves and add,
conserve or consume resources.
Decide on course of action to realise
creative potential for self.

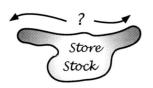

Distribution and Storage
**Gall Bladder and
Liver**

NOURISHMENT
Need for nourishment.
Amoeba asserts its desire via
pseudopodium and engulfs food
and digestion follows.
The hunger created by the need
is satisfied.

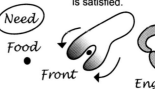

Ingestion and Digestion
**Stomach and
Spleen**

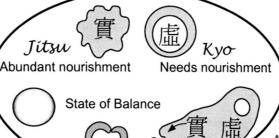

Jitsu
Abundant nourishment

Kyo
Needs nourishment

State of Balance

PROTECTION
Protect boundaries
against environmental or
social agents.
Extends self centre towards
or away from social environment or
community hence sharing and communicating.

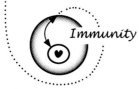

Circulation and Protection
**Heart Governor and
Triple Heater**

CONTROL
Absorb into and make part of self.
Absorption of nourishment
including ideas, emotions and nutrients.
Maintain presence and awareness
to experience life.

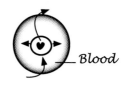

Integration and Conversion
**Heart and
Small Intestine**

IMPETUS
Moving away from threats
in the environment in order to
survive or find safety.
Propulsion or impetus of body
activities helps purify
thus prevent stagnation.

Purification and Impetus
**Bladder and
Kidney**

" Meridians and movement of protoplasm in a single celled organism are the same thing called by different names. We regard amoebas as also having meridians since amoebas live by movement of protoplasm and exist as independant living entities. Amoebas perform the basic life functions of locomotion, ingestion, elimination and reproduction and are also capable of defensive reactions like higher forms of life such as human beings. All these basic life functions depend on the working of the meridians. This implies that the movement of Ki, which sustains life, is revealed in an observable form by the structure and movement of the body."
Shizuto Masunaga,
'Zen Imagery Exercises', p59, Japan Publications, 1987

Fig. 2.17 Zen Shiatsu: Basic Kyo (虚) - Jitsu (實) modes and Tsubo (壺) types

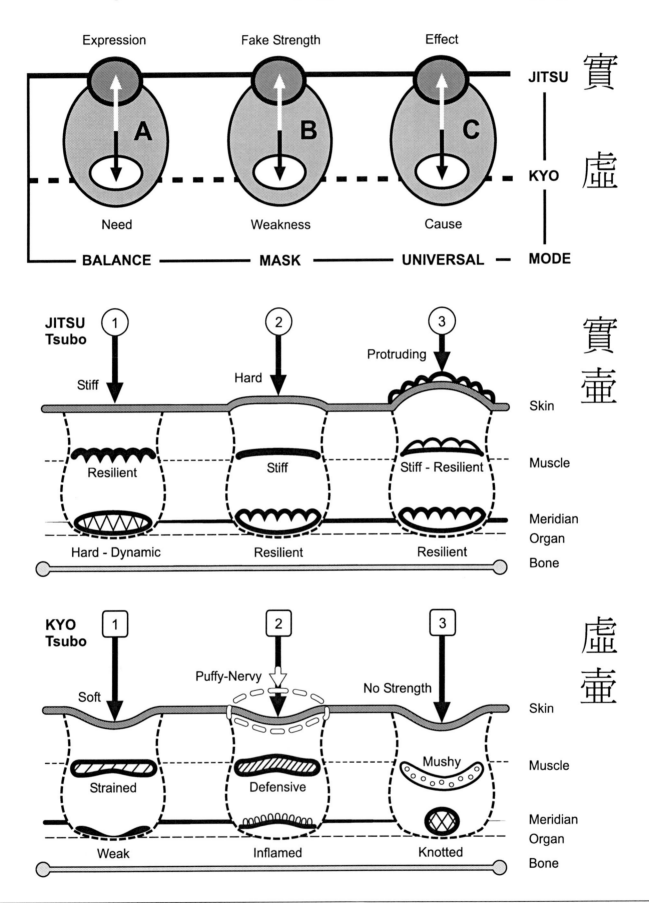

** After Pauline Sasaki and Clifford Andrews, Grimstone Manor, England 1990. **

Chapter 3
YIN-YANG primary vessels

Controller
and
Supervisor vessels

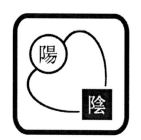

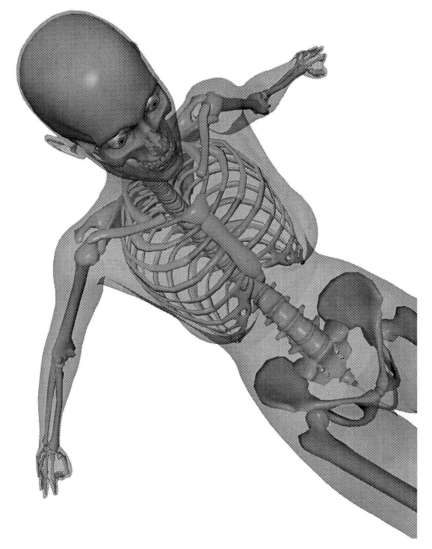

Fig. 3.1 Tai Ji and Primary vessels: Cosmological creation sequence

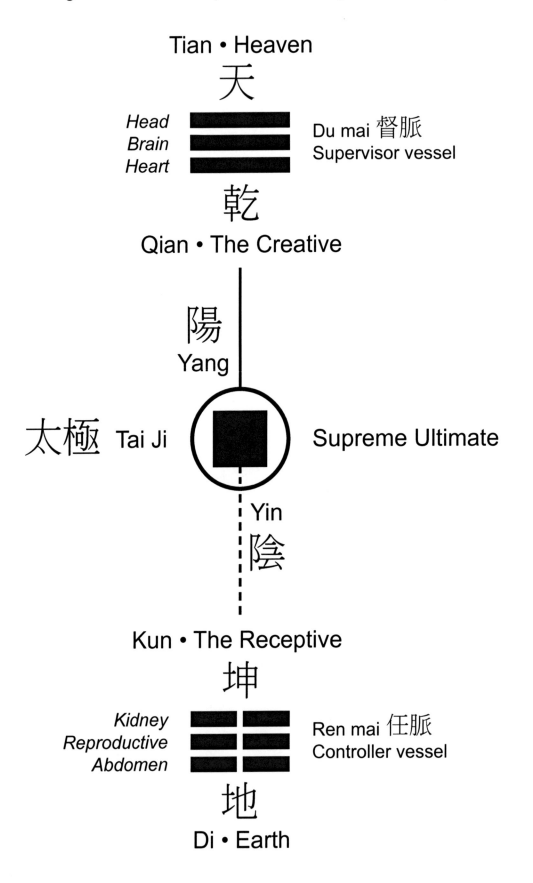

Supervisor Vessel Points • Du Mai Xue • 督脈穴

IDENTIFICATION	ACTION	INDICATIONS
SV-1 Changqiang 長強 Lasting Strength Located midway between the tip of the COCCYX and the ANUS. *Luo-CONNECTING POINT of the Supervisor vessel* *MEETING POINT of the Supervisor vessel with the Controller vessel and the Gall Bladder and Kidney channels*	Regulates the Supervisor and Controller vessels Resolves Damp Heat Calms the Mind	Back pain, fatigue Haemorrhoids Hysteria, hypomania
SV-2 Yaoshu 腰俞 Lumbar Shu On the posterior midline, in the SACRO-COCCYGEAL hiatus.	Strengthens Lower Back Expels Interior Wind and Damp	Lower back and sacral pain radiating down leg to foot Epilepsy Chills and stiffness of hips Irregular menstruation Haemorrhoids
SV-4 Mingmen 命門 Gate of Life Located inferior to the SPINOUS process of the 2nd LUMBAR VERTEBRA, in a depression on the posterior midline.	Tonifies Kidney Yang (c/w Moxibustion) (caution if Heat symptoms anywhere) Nourishes Original Qi Benefits Essence Strengthens Lower Back Expels Cold (Yang deficiency)	Fatigue, chilliness, abundant clear urination, depression, weakness of legs, pale tongue Chronic physical and mental weakness, reproductive disorders Chronic lumbar stiffness or pain Chronic diarrhoea, intestinal pain, incontinence, reproductive disorders
SV-14 Dazhui 大椎 Great Vertebra Located inferior to the SPINOUS process of the 7th CERVICAL VERTEBRA, on the posterior midline. *MEETING POINT of the Supervisor vessel with the Six Yang channels of the Hand and Foot* *SEA of QI POINT*	Releases the Exterior Expels Wind Clears Heat Regulates Nutritive and Defensive Qi Calms the Mind Stimulates the Brain	Asthma, common cold, fullness of chest Neck and spinal stiffness and pain Fever and chills Epilepsy Hay fever and eczema, sweating Mania, hysteria, headache Unclear thinking
SV-16 Fengfu 風府 Wind Palace In the depression directly inferior to the OCCIPITAL PROTRUBERANCE, on the posterior midline, approximately 1 CUN above the hairline on the nape of the NECK. *MEETING POINT of the Supervisor vessel and Yin Tie vessel* *SEA of MARROW POINT* *Sun Si-miao GHOST POINT*	Regulates the Supervisor and Controller vessels Resolves Damp Heat Calms the Mind	Back pain, fatigue Haemorrhoids Hysteria, hypomania

Supervisor Vessel Points • Du Mai Xue • 督脈穴

IDENTIFICATION	ACTION	INDICATIONS
SV-20 Bahui 百會 Hundred Meetings Located on the cranial midline of the HEAD, in the hollow 8 CUN posterior to the GLABELLA and 6 CUN superior to the vertex of the EXTERNAL OCCIPITAL PROTUBERANCE (INION). Alternatively locate 5 CUN posterior to the frontal hairline and 7 CUN superior to the posterior hairline. *MEETING POINT of the Supervisor vessel with the Bladder, Gall Bladder, Triple Heater and Liver channels* *SEA of MARROW POINT* **** Moxibustion contra-indicated if high blood pressure or heat symptoms ****	Calms the Mind Tonifies Yang (c/w Moxibustion) Strengthens Spleen ascending function Promotes resuscitation c/w SV-26 Renzhong & HG-6 Neiguan	Unclear thinking, depression Prolapse of Stomach Prolapse of Bladder Prolapse of Uterus Prolapse of Anus Prolapse of Vagina Haemorrhoids Unconsciousness
SV-26 Renzhong 人中 Person's Middle Located on the PHILTRUM about one third the distance from the base of the NOSE to the tip of the LIP. *MEETING POINT of the Supervisor vessel with the Stomach and Large Intestine channels* *Sun Si-miao GHOST POINT* **** Moxibustion is contra-indicated ****	Promotes resuscitation Benefits Lumbar Spine	Unconsciousness, drowsiness Acute lower back sprain
SV-28 Yinjiao 齦交 Gum Intersection At the junction of the upper LIP and GUM, on the SUPERIOR FRENULUM inside the MOUTH. *MEETING POINT of the Supervisor vessel and the Controller vessel*	Resolves Damp Heat	Painful swollen gums Haemorrhoids

Controller Vessel Points • Ren Mai Xue • 任脈穴

IDENTIFICATION	ACTION	INDICATIONS
CV-1 Huiyin 會陰 Meeting of Yin Located at the centre of the PERINEUM, midway between the ANUS and the SCROTUM in males, and between the ANUS and POSTERIOR LABIAL COMMISSURE in females. *MEETING POINT of the Controller vessel, Through-way vessel and the Supervisor vessel* *Sun Si-miao GHOST POINT*	Nourishes Yin Stabilises Essence Resolves Damp Heat Restores consciousness	Incontinence Reproductive disorders Genital or perineal pain, itching or swelling Cessation of breathing due to near drowning
CV-3 Zhongji 中極 Central Pole 4 CUN inferior to the UMBILICUS on the anterior midline and 1 CUN superior to the PUBIC SYMPHYSIS. *FRONT Mu-COLLECTING POINT of the Bladder* *MEETING POINT of the Controller vessel with the Spleen, Liver and Kidney channels* **** Contra-indicated during pregnancy ****	Regulates Bladder Resolves Damp Heat Clears Heat	Urinary incontinence or retention Pain and burning on urination Inflammation of Bladder (Cystitis) Genital pain or itching Blood in urine, burning urination
CV-4 Guanyuan 関元 Origin Pass 3 CUN inferior to the UMBILICUS on the anterior midline and 2 CUN superior to the PUBIC SYMPHYSIS. *FRONT Mu-COLLECTING POINT of the Small Intestine* *MEETING POINT of the Controller vessel with the Spleen, Liver and Kidney channels* **** Contra-indicated during pregnancy ****	Nourishes Blood and Yin Regulates the Uterus Tonifies the Kidneys Benefits Original Qi Tonifies Yang (with Moxibustion) Regulates Small Intestine Roots Ethereal Soul (the Hun)	Severe anxiety, absence or scanty menstruation and uterine disorders Infertility Asthma Urinary disorders due to chronic fatigue or constitutional weakness Pain and weakness of the lower back, bones and joints of the legs particularly in the elderly or middle- aged Chronic fatigue or weakness with cold extremities Diarrhoea Vague feeling of fear at night

Controller Vessel Points • Ren Mai Xue • 任脈穴

IDENTIFICATION	ACTION	INDICATIONS
CV-5 Shimen 石門 Stone Gate 2 CUN inferior to the UMBILICUS on the anterior midline, and 1 CUN superior to the PUBIC SYMPHYSIS. *FRONT Mu-COLLECTING POINT of the Triple Heater* **** Contra-indicated during pregnancy ****	Tonifies Original Qi Regulates fluids in Lower Heater	Kidney deficiency Poor constitution Abdominal oedema Urinary retention or incontinence Diarrhoea Vaginal discharge
CV-6 Qihai 氣海 Sea of Qi 1.5 CUN inferior to the UMBILICUS on the anterior midline, and 3.5 CUN superior to the PUBIC SYMPHYSIS. **** Contra-indicated during pregnancy ****	Tonifies Qi and Yang (c/w Moxibustion) Tonifies Original Qi (c/w Moxibustion) Resolves Dampness (Lower Heater) Regulates Qi	Extreme physical and mental exhaustion and depression Fatigue, loose stools, chills, abundant pale urination, depression and lack of willpower Vaginal discharge or loose stools with mucus, difficult urination Stagnancy, pain or distension in the lower abdomen
CV-8 Shenque 神闕 Spirit Gateway Located in the centre of the UMBILICUS. **** Acupuncture contra-indicated ****	Tonifies Yang Tonifies and strengthens the Spleen (Use with indirect Moxibustion after filling Umbilicus with salt)	Extreme fatigue and internal cold Chronic diarrhoea
CV-12 Zhongwan 中脘 Middle Cavity 4 CUN superior to the UMBILICUS on the anterior midline, midway between the STERNOCOSTAL angle and the UMBILICUS. *FRONT Mu-COLLECTING POINT of the Stomach* *FRONT COLLECTING POINT of the Middle Heater* *Hui-MEETING POINT of the Fu (six yang organs)* *MEETING POINT of the Controller vessel with the Small Intestine, Triple Heater and Stomach channels*	Tonifies Stomach and Spleen (c/w Moxibustion for Cold) Resolves Dampness	Lack of appetite, digestive weakness, tiredness with cold Abdominal distension and pain Constipation with headache General feeling of heaviness

Controller Vessel Points • Ren Mai Xue • 任脈穴

IDENTIFICATION	ACTION	INDICATIONS
CV-14 Juque 巨闕 Great Gateway 6 CUN superior to the UMBILICUS on the anterior midline, 2 CUN inferior to the STERNOCOSTAL angle. *FRONT Mu-COLLECTING POINT of the Heart*	Subdues rebellious Stomach Qi Calms the Mind Clears the Heart	Mental anxiety, heartburn, vomiting, regurgitation, hiccups, difficulty in swallowing (mainly due to emotional origin) Forgetfulness, fearful palpitations, anxiety
CV-17 Shanzong / Tanzhong 膻中 Thorax Centre On the anterior midline, level with the junction of the 4th INTERCOSTAL SPACE with the STERNUM, and between the NIPPLES. *FRONT Mu-COLLECTING POINT of the Heart Governor* *FRONT Mu-COLLECTING POINT of the Upper Heater* *Hui-MEETING POINT of the QI* *SEA of QI POINT* *MEETING POINT of the Controller vessel with the Spleen, Kidney, Small Intestine and Triple Heater channels*	Tonifies Qi Regulates Qi Resolves Phlegm Facilitates Lactation	Breathlessness, bronchitis, asthma, lack of vitality with pale face, cough, chest pain, palpitations, intercostal neuralgia, hiccups, anxiety Cough, chronic bronchitis Insufficient lactation
CV-22 Tiantu 天突 Heaven's Chimney Located at the SUPRASTERNAL FOSSA 0.5 SUN above the STERNAL NOTCH	Descends Lung Qi Resolves Phlegm Clears Heat	Acute and chronic asthma and cough Acute bronchitis with profuse sputum, lung and throat mucus Sore throat due to exterior pathogen (Wind-Heat)
CV-24 Chengjiang 承漿 Container of Tears Superior to the CHIN, in the depression at the centre of the MENTOLABIAL GROOVE. *MEETING POINT of the Controller vessel with the Supervisor vessel and the Large Intestine and Stomach channels* *Sun Si-miao GHOST POINT*	Expels Exterior Wind	Paralysis of the face and mouth

Table 3.1 The Primary vessels correspondences: Supervisor vessel (Du mai)

SUPERVISOR vessel		Du mai 督脈
FACULTY	Spiritual Input	: Yuan-Shen: Shen, Spirit-Mind
	Functions via	: Conciousness
	Represents	: Spatial Awareness
	Supplemented by	: Nervous Centre
		: Yuan Qi: Ministerial Fire
	Realised by	: Initiating and Relaying
	Dominant Zone	: Head, Eyes, Back, Shoulders
	Embryological Layer	: Ectoderm
	Meridian Nature	: Yang
	Tuning Time	: 3am (between Liver and Lung)
ANATOMY & PHYSIOLOGY	Brain	] Central Nervous System (CNS)
	Cerebrum, Cerebellum	] Autonomic Nervous System (ANS)
	Medulla Oblongata, Pons	]
	Pituitary and Pineal glands	]
	Posterior Hypothalamus	] Senso-Physical Initiative
	Spinal cord	] Information, Movement, and
	Eyes	] Balance Response
	Nose and Tongue	] Taste
	Heart, Sino-atrial Node	] Circulatory system
	Atrio-ventricular node	]
	Clitoris, Ovaries, Penis, Prostate	] Hormonal System
	gland, Testes, Uterus, Sex	] Reproductive System
	chromosomes X+Y and Sperm	]
PHYSICAL	Absence of Menses	Intestinal Disorders inc Rectal/Anal
	Asthma	Neck and Back Pain
	Colds, Sneezing	Nasal Problems
	Dizziness	Night sweating
	Eczema	Palpitations
	Eye, Nose and Throat Problems	Paralysis of hands and feet
	Fever	Opisthotonos
	Haemorrhoids	Seminal Emission, Discharges
	Headaches	Spasms inc Epileptic Seizures
	Infertility	Urogenital Disorders
PSYCHOLOGICAL	Anxiety	Manic-depressive
	Dementia	Memory Loss
	Disorganised	Mental Problems
	Emotional Irritability	Loss of Consciousness
	Halluciations	Overactive
	Hypersensitive	Relationship and Sexual Problems
	Hypomania	Sensitive to Extreme Change
	Insomnia	Unclear Thinking
	Mania	Vertigo
SUPERVISOR vessel		Du mai 督脈

Table 3.2 The Primary vessels correspondences: Controller vessel (Ren mai)

CONTROLLER vessel		Ren mai 任脈
FACULTY	Spiritual Input	: Yuan Shen: Po, Corporeal Soul
	Functions via	: Physical Body
	Represents	: Material Awareness
	Supplemented by	: Reproductive Organs
		: Yuan Qi: Essence
	Realised by	: Nourishing and Completing
	Dominant Zone	: Abdomen, Chest, Throat/Mouth
	Embryological Layer	: Endoderm, Mesoderm
	Meridian Nature	: Yin
	Tuning Time	: 3am (between Liver and Lung)
ANATOMY & PHYSIOLOGY	Anterior Hypothalamus	] Hormonal System (EGS)
	Pituitary gland, Eyes	] Senso-Physical Initiative
	Mouth, Oesophagus	] Digestive and Respiratory Systems
	Throat, Lungs and Heart	] Blood Quality and Regulation
	Small and Large Intestines	]
	Liver, Kidney and Placenta	]
	Breasts, Cervix, Clitoris,	] Hormonal System
	Ova (mature egg), Ovaries,	] Reproductive System
	Penis, Prostate gland, Sex	]
	chromosome X, Spermatozoa,	]
	Testes, Uterus, Vagina and	]
	Zygote (fertilized egg)	]
PHYSICAL	Acne, Eczema	Hernia
	Asthma	Heart Problems
	Constipation	Infertility
	Cough	Labour Difficulties
	Chest and Throat Problems	Menopausal Syndromes
	Diabetes	Menstrual Problems
	Diarrhoea	Mouth, Gum, Teeth Problems
	Epilepsy	Pain of Abdomen, Chest, Throat
	Extreme Fatigue, Exhaustion	Oedema
	Headaches	Urinary and Uterine Disorders
PSYCHOLOGICAL	Agitated	Forgetfulness
	Anger	Loss of Consciousness
	Anxiety	Manic-depressive
	Burdened, Duty Bound	Mood Swings
	Confidence Issues	Over Mothering
	Depression	Post-Partum Depression
	Emotional Trauma	Protective Attitude
	Excessive Sighing	Relationship and Sexual Problems
	Fear (vague sense of at night)	Social Difficulties
	Frightful Palpitations	Territorial Issues

Fig. 3.2 Anterior view of the Controller (Ren mai) and Supervisor (Du mai) vessels

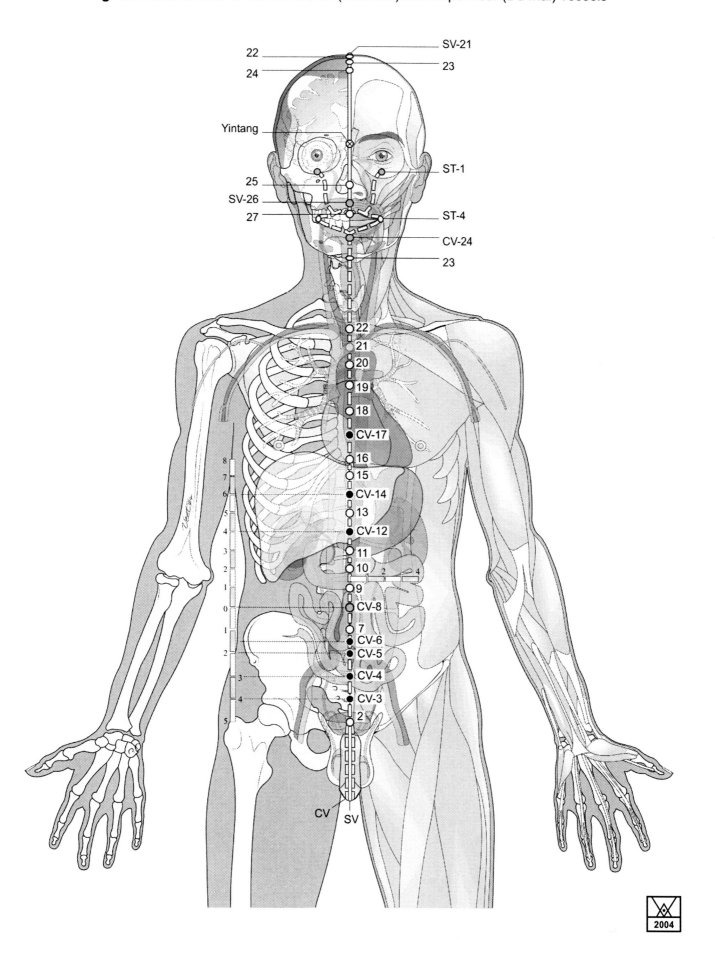

Fig. 3.3 Posterior view of the Supervisor (Du mai) and Controller (Ren mai) vessels

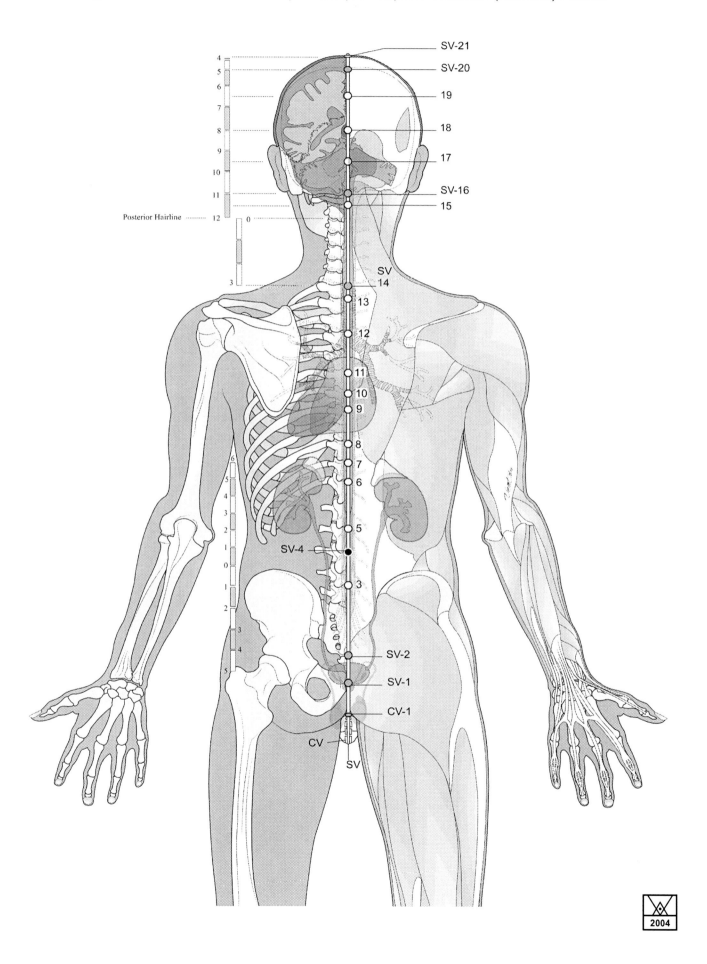

Fig. 3.4 Head: cranial and lateral details of the Supervisor (Du mai)) and Controller (Ren mai) vessels

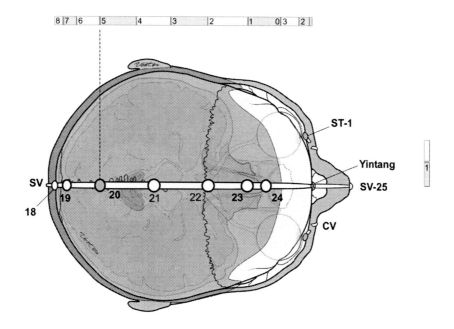

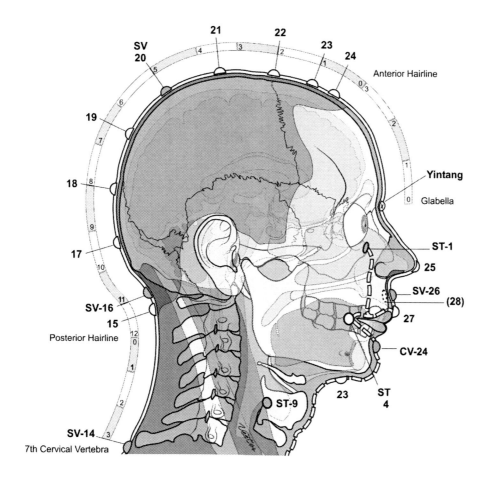

Fig. 3.5 Male perineum details: Supervisor (Du mai) and Controller (Ren mai) vessels

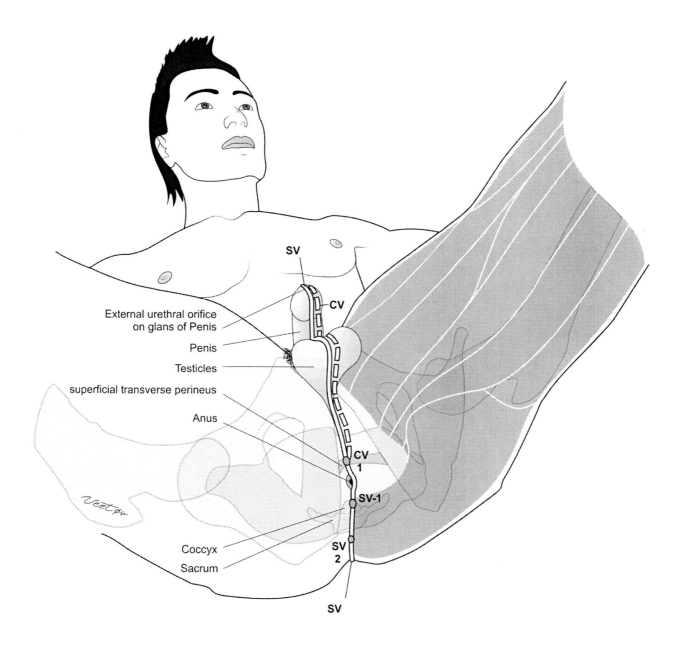

SV

CV

External urethral orifice
on glans of Penis

Penis

Testicles

superficial transverse perineus

Anus

CV
1

SV-1

Coccyx

SV
2

Sacrum

SV

2004

Fig. 3.6 Female perineum details: Supervisor (Du mai) and Controller (Ren mai) vessels

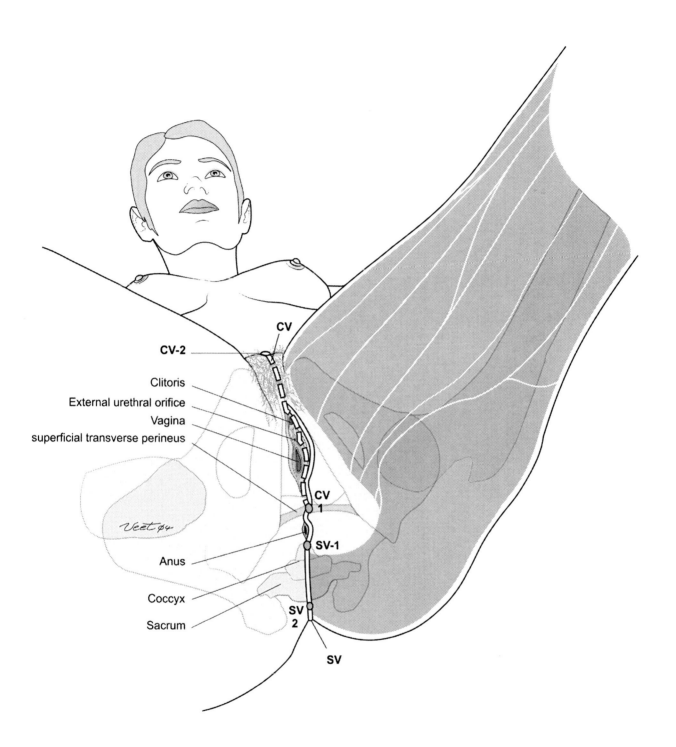

Chapter 4
the WATER element

Bladder
and
Kidneys

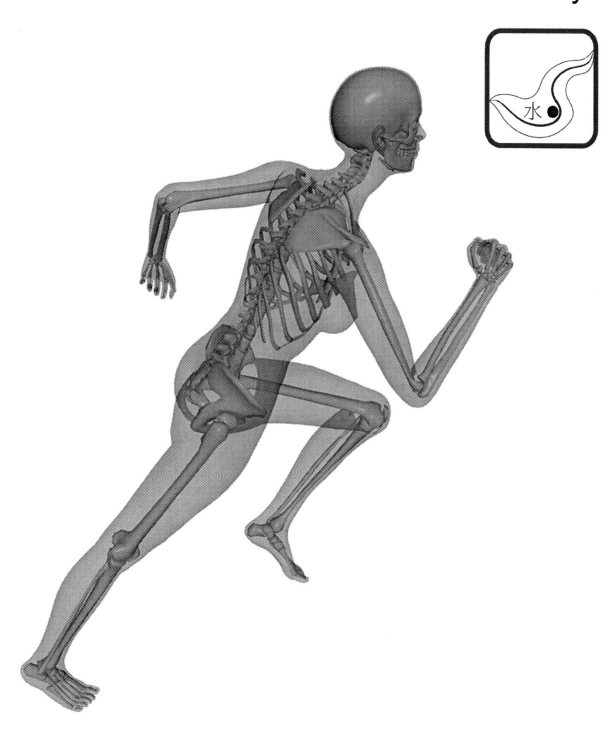

Fig. 4.1 The Five element sequences: WATER

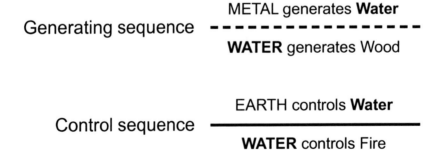

Fire

Wood

Earth

WATER

Metal

Generating sequence	METAL generates **Water**
	– – – – – – – – – – – – –
	WATER generates Wood

Control sequence	EARTH controls **Water**
	————————
	WATER controls Fire

Table 4.1 The Five element correspondences: WATER

The WATER element		Shui xing 水行
FACULTY	Spiritual	: Zhi, Will
		Jing, Essence
	Celestial Stems	: Ren (stem 9) and Gui (stem 10)
	Earthly branches	: Hai (branch 12) and Zi (branch 1)
	Planet	: Mercury
	Number	: 6
	Pentatonic note	: Yu, (Mi, 3rd note of scale)
	Genetic aspiration	: Conception via procreation and survival
	Cycle	: Storage
	Yin/Yang	: Utmost Yin
	Quality	: Floating
ENVIRONMENTAL	Season	: Winter
	Phase of Moon	: Half moon decreasing to black moon
	Climate	: Cold
	Direction	: North
	Colour	: Black
	Part of the Day	: Night
BODY	Organ Yin	: Kidneys
	Yang	: Bladder
	Tissue	: Marrow, Bones
	Skin Colour	: Black, Blue
	Odour	: Putrid
	Branch	: Head Hair
	Sense Organ	: Ears
	Senses	: Hearing
	Fluid	: Watery Saliva, Urine
EMOTIONAL	Emotion	: Fear, Courage
	Sound, Voice	: Groaning, Humming
	Action	: Trembling
FOOD (symbol)	Animal	: Pig, Fish
	Taste	: Salty
	Fruit	: Chestnut
	Grain	: Beans
	Vegetable	: Root plants (cabbages, kale, mushrooms)

Bladder Channel Points • Pang Guang Jing Xue • 膀胱經穴

IDENTIFICATION	ACTION	INDICATIONS
BL-1 Jingming 精明 Eye Brightness Near the medial ORBITAL BORDER, lateral and 0.1 CUN superior to the INNER CANTHUS. *MEETING POINT of the Small Intestine, Triple Heater, Stomach, and Bladder channels with the Supervisor vessel, Yin Walker vessel and the Yang Walker vessel* **** Moxibustion is contra-indicated ****	Expels Exterior Wind Clears Heat	All eye problems including red, painful, swollen and dry eyes Frontal and occipital headaches Dizziness Colour or night blindness Pituitary, Hypothalamus and Pineal gland problems
BL-2 Zanzhu 攢竹 Gathering Bamboo In the hollow at the medial end of the EYEBROW in the SUPRAORBITAL NOTCH	Expels Wind Brightens Eyes Soothes Liver Removes Channel obstructions Clears the Nose	Facial paralysis and tics Trigeminal Neuralgia Red eyes, blurred vision Eye problems where other Liver distortions are present Frontal headaches and pain around or behind eyes Lower back problems Sinusitis, Rhinitis and Hay Fever
BL-10 Tianzhu 天柱 Heavens Pillar 1.3 CUN lateral to SV-15 Yamen, on the lateral border of the TRAPEZIUS muscle. *SEA of QI POINT*	Expels Interior and Exterior Wind Clears the Brain Brightens the Eyes Removes Channel obstructions	Occipital and vertical type headaches Stiff neck, nasal congestion Memory and concentration problems Dim vision, eye pain Back pain, neck injuries Cold type pain with stiffness
BL-11 Dazhu 大杼 Great Shuttle 1.5 CUN lateral to the centre of the SPINE between the 1st and 2nd THORACIC VERTEBRA. *SEA of BLOOD POINT, Hui-MEETING POINT of the BONES MEETING POINT of the Bladder and Small Intestine channels*	Strengthens the Bones and Joints Regulates Lung Qi Releases the Exterior Expels wind Soothes the Sinews	Pain and stiffness of the neck, spine, scapula and knees Promotes bone growth in children Prevents degeneration of bone in the elderly Cough, chest pain and fullness Cold, fever and chills, muscular ache, headache, dizziness Contraction of the tendons

Bladder Channel Points • Pang Guang Jing Xue • 膀胱經穴

IDENTIFICATION	ACTION	INDICATIONS
BL-13 Feishu 肺俞 Lung Shu 1.5 CUN lateral to the centre of the SPINE between the 3rd and 4th THORACIC VERTEBRA *BACK Shu-TRANSPORTING POINT of the Lung*	Stimulates the Lung Dispersing/Descending function Clears Interior Heat Tonifies Lung Qi Regulates Lung Defensive Qi	Cough due to Exterior pattern Asthma, cough or breathless symptoms due to Interior pattern Acute Heat conditions i.e. high fever, thirst, cough, breathlessness, sticky yellow sputum, restlessness Breathlessness, chest pain, tight chest, neck or back pain Grief or sadness Skin problems, sweating and fever
BL-14 Jueyinshu 厥陰俞 Absolute Yin Shu 1.5 CUN lateral to the centre of the SPINE between the 4th and 5th THORACIC VERTEBRA. *BACK Shu-TRANSPORTING POINT of the Heart Governor*	Regulates the Heart Calms the Mind	Heartbeat problems, pain Coronary heart disease Anxiety and restlessness
BL-15 Xinshu 心俞 Heart Shu 1.5 CUN lateral to the centre of the SPINE between the 5th and 6th THORACIC VERTEBRA. *BACK Shu-TRANSPORTING POINT of the Heart*	Clears Heat Calms the Mind Stimulates the Brain Invigorates the Blood	Nervous anxiety and insomnia Night sweats Heat in palms and soles Excess conditions of the Heart Concentration and memory problems Heart or chest pain due to stasis of blood
BL-16 Dushu 督俞 Supervisor Shu 1.5 CUN lateral to the centre of the SPINE between the 6th and 7th THORACIC VERTEBRA *BACK Shu-TRANSPORTING POINT of the Supervisor vessel*	Regulates the Heart Invigorates the Blood	Heart or chest pain Removes blood stasis

Bladder Channel Points • Pang Guang Jing Xue • 膀胱經穴

IDENTIFICATION	ACTION	INDICATIONS
BL-17 Geshu 膈俞 Diaphragm Shu 1.5 CUN lateral to the centre of the SPINE between the 7th and 8th THORACIC VERTEBRA. *DIAPHRAGM Shu or BACK TRANSPORTING POINT* *HUI-MEETING POINT of the BLOOD*	Nourishes Blood and Qi c/w direct Moxibustion Invigorates the Blood Removes obstruction from the Diaphragm Pacifies Stomach Qi	Absence of menses Blood deficiency of organs (treat BL 17 c/w relevant SHU point) Lethargy Dizziness Blood stasis in organs or any part of the body Chest pain, hiccup, belching Hiccup, belching, nausea and vomiting
BL-18 Ganshu 肝俞 Liver Shu 1.5 CUN lateral to the centre of the SPINE between the 9th and 10th THORACIC VERTEBRA. *BACK Shu-TRANSPORTING POINT* *of the Liver*	Moves stagnant Qi Resolves Damp Heat Benefits the Eyes Tonifies Liver Blood	Distension of epigastrium and hypochondrium Sour regurgitation and nausea Jaundice and inflammation of the Gall Bladder Poor night vision, blurred eyes Red, painful eyes Fatigue Atrophy syndrome (wasting)
BL-19 Danshu 膽俞 Gall Bladder Shu 1.5 CUN lateral to the centre of the SPINE between the 10th and 11th THORACIC VERTEBRA. *BACK Shu-TRANSPORTING POINT* *of the Gall Bladder*	Resolves Damp Heat Pacifies Stomach Qi Relaxes Diaphragm	Inflammation of Gall Bladder Jaundice Inflammation of Pancreas Nausea, belching, vomiting and heartburn Hiccup Full feeling under the diaphragm due to stagnation of Liver Qi
BL-20 Pishu 脾俞 Spleen Shu 1.5 CUN lateral to the centre of the SPINE between the 11th and 12th THORACIC VERTEBRA. *BACK Shu-TRANSPORTING POINT* *of the Spleen*	Tonifies Spleen and Stomach Resolves Damp Nourishes Blood	Tiredness, loose stools, no appetite Abdominal distension Prolapse of Stomach Prolapse of Uterus Asthma, Oedema on torso Dizziness and vertigo Anaemia Mental exhaustion, chronic fatigue

Bladder Channel Points • Pang Guang Jing Xue • 膀胱經穴

IDENTIFICATION	ACTION	INDICATIONS
BL-21 Weishu 胃俞 Stomach Shu 1.5 CUN lateral to the centre of the SPINE between the 12th THORACIC VERTEBRA and the 1st LUMBAR VERTEBRA. *BACK Shu-TRANSPORTING POINT of the Stomach*	Tonifies Stomach and Spleen Resolves Damp Pacifies Stomach	Loss of appetite Stomach pain, Epigastric pain Pain in the chest or in hypochondriac zone Asthma, oedema, dizziness and vertigo Belching, hiccup, nausea and vomiting Retention of food causing bloating and regurgitation of food Difficulty swallowing
BL-22 Sanjiaoshu 三焦俞 Triple Heater Shu 1.5 CUN lateral to the centre of the SPINE between the 1st and 2nd LUMBAR VERTEBRA. *BACK Shu-TRANSPORTING POINT of the Triple Heater*	Resolves Dampness Opens Water Passages	Urinary retention Painful urination Oedema of legs Fluid problems in lower torso Kidney stones Lower back pain
BL-23 Shenshu 腎俞 Kidney Shu 1.5 CUN lateral to the centre of the SPINE between the 2nd and 3rd LUMBAR VERTEBRA. *BACK Shu-TRANSPORTING POINT of the Kidneys*	Tonifies Kidneys Nourishes Essence Strengthens Kidney function of receiving Qi Strengthens Lower Back Benefits Bones and Marrow Benefits Ears and Eyes Nourishes Blood Resolves Dampness	Chronic fatigue, tiredness Lack of willpower Impotence, infertility, lack of sexual desire Excessive urination Chilling in lower body Chronic Asthma Chronic lower backache Arthritic bone deformities Dizziness Poor memory Weak legs Tinnitus, deafness Chronic eye disorders, poor vision, dry eyes Anaemia Menstrual syndromes: absence of menses; irregular menstruation; menstrual pain Fullness of Bladder, with feeling of distension Urinary stones

Bladder Channel Points • Pang Guang Jing Xue • 膀胱經穴

IDENTIFICATION	ACTION	INDICATIONS
BL-25 Dachangshu 大腸俞 Large Intestine Shu 1.5 CUN lateral to the the centre of the SPINE between the 4th and 5th LUMBAR VERTEBRA *BACK Shu-TRANSPORTING POINT of the Large Intestine*	Promotes Large Intestine function Strengthens Lower Back	Constipation, diarrhoea, flatulence Chronic Large Intestine disease: Diverticulitis Colitis Abdominal fullness, distension Rectal prolapse Acute/chronic backache Sciatica Stiffness
BL-27 Xiaochangshu 小腸俞 Small Intestine Shu 1.5 CUN lateral to the centre of the SACRAL SPINE, level with the 1st SACRAL FORAMEN. *BACK Shu-TRANSPORTING POINT of the Small intestine*	Promotes Small Intestine function Resolves Dampness Lower Heater	Abdominal pain, intestinal rumbling Mucus in stools Diarrhoea Cloudy and difficult urination Inflammation of Bladder (Cystitis)
BL-28 Pangguanshu 膀胱俞 Bladder Shu 1.5 CUN lateral to the centre of the SACRAL SPINE, level with the 2nd SACRAL FORAMEN. *BACK Shu-TRANSPORTING POINT of the Bladder*	Regulates Bladder Clears Heat/Dampness Lower Heater Opens Water Passages Strengthens Lower Back	Urinary incontinence Urination with seminal discharge Urinary tract infection Blood in the urine Inflammation of Prostate Gland Burning urination Oedema, Frequent urination Sacroiliac pain or stiffness, Sciatica Coldness in lower body or pelvis Lower back or pelvic pain
BL-36 Chengfu 承扶 Hold and Support Below the buttock, at the midpoint of the transverse GLUTEAL crease, between theTENDONS of the BICEPS FEMORIS and SEMITENDINOSUS muscles.	Strengthens Lower Back and lower limbs Regulates the Lower Heater	Sciatica (lower backache with pain radiating down the back of the leg) Pain in lumbar, sacral, coccyx and gluteal areas Chronic and bleeding haemorrhoids, Constipation Pain in genitals, urinary problems, seminal emission and cold in uterus

Bladder Channel Points • Pang Guang Jing Xue • 膀胱經穴

IDENTIFICATION	ACTION	INDICATIONS
BL-40 Weizhong 委中 Middle of the Crook Mid point of the transverse crease of the POPLITEAL FOSSA located between the TENDONS of the BICEPS FEMORIS and SEMITENDINOSUS muscles. *He-SEA POINT of the Bladder channel* *EARTH POINT of the Bladder channel* *Ma Dan-yang HEAVENLY STAR POINT* **** Use Moxibustion with caution ****	Removes Channel obstructions Resolves Dampness Cools Blood Clears Heat Eliminates Blood stasis	Acute backache Sciatica Burning urination Skin diseases of a heat nature: Herpes Zoster Fever and delirium Varicose veins Lower leg pain
BL-43 Gaohuangshu 膏肓俞 Fatty Vital Shu 3 CUN lateral to the centre of the SPINE between the 4th and 5th THORACIC VERTEBRA and level with BL-14 Jueyinshu (approximately level with the spinous process of the 4th thoracic vertebra).	Tonifies Qi and Strengthens Deficiency (use MOXA) Nourish Essence Nourishes Lung Yin Invigorates the Mind	Chronic illnessess, night sweating disorders Emaciation Impotence, seminal emission also with dreams Chronic Lung disease, asthma, bronchitis, dry cough Poor memory, insomnia
BL-52 Zhishi 志室 Will Chamber 3 CUN lateral to the centre of the SPINE between the 2nd and 3rd LUMBAR VERTEBRA (approximately level with the spinous process of the 2nd lumbar vertebra).	Tonifies the Kidneys Strenghtens the Back Reinforces the Zhi (Willpower)	Impotence, seminal emission also with dreams, pain and swelling of the genitals and perineum Urinary problems Chronic lower back pain Depression and disoriented thinking

Bladder Channel Points • Pang Guang Jing Xue • 膀胱經穴

IDENTIFICATION	ACTION	INDICATIONS
BL-57 Chengsan 承山 Supporting Mountain 8 CUN below BL-40 Weizhong, inferior to the belly of the GASTROCNEMIUS muscle on a line connecting BL-40 Weizhong to the ACHILLES TENDON. *Ma Dan-yang HEAVENLY STAR POINT*	Strengthens Lower Back Relaxes Tendons including Ligaments Invigorates Blood	Lower backache Sciatica Cramping of the Gastrocnemius muscle Menstrual pain Blood in the stools Haemorrhoids, varicose veins Rectal prolapse
BL-60 Kunlun 崑崙 Kunlun Mountains Between the posterior border of the LATERAL MALLEOLUS and the medial aspect of the ACHILLES TENDON, level with the vertex of the LATERAL MALLEOLUS *Jing-RIVER POINT* *FIRE POINT of the Bladder channel* **** Contra-indicated during pregnancy ****	Strengthens the Lower Back Painful obstruction on Channel Disperses Internal and External Wind Expedites Labour Clears Heat	Chronic backache presenting in deficiency pattern Shoulder, neck and occipital pain or stiffness Sciatica Ankle/heel pain Difficult labour Burning urination
BL-67 Zhiyin 至陰 Reaching Yin About 0.1 CUN from the lateral corner of the 5th TOENAIL, level with the base line of the nail. *Jing-WELL POINT* *METAL POINT of the Bladder channel* **** Contra-indicated during pregnancy except as indicated ****	Eliminates Internal and External Wind Calms Foetus Used at 8th month of pregnancy with MOXA Expedites Labour	Headaches Nasal congestion and discharge Blurred and painful eyes Breech presentation (malposition of foetus) Difficult labour

Kidney Channel Points • Shen Jing Xue • 腎經穴

IDENTIFICATION	ACTION	INDICATIONS
KD-1 Yongquan 湧泉 Gushing Spring In a depression on the sole when the FOOT is plantar flexed, one third the distance from a line between the base of the 2nd and 3rd TOES and the back centre of the HEEL. *Jing-WELL POINT* *WOOD POINT of the Kidney channel*	Tonifies Yin Calms the Mind Clears Fire and Heat Subdues Wind	Infertility Oedema Kidney and back pain Sensation of heat in the soles of the feet Extreme fear, insomnia, severe anxiety Shock, mental illness Loss of consciousness Dizziness, epilepsy High blood pressure Headaches presenting at the top of the head
KD-3 Taixi 太谿 Supreme Ravine Midway between the MEDIAL MALLEOLUS and the ACHILLES TENDON level with the vertex of the MEDIAL MALLEOLUS. *Yuan-SOURCE POINT* *Shu-STREAM POINT* *EARTH POINT of the Kidney channel*	Tonifies the Kidneys and Essence Strengthens Original Qi Regulates the Uterus Strengthens the Lower Back and Knees	Chronic tiredness Impotence Tinnitus Urinary dysfunction Kidney inflammation Lack of willpower Bone problems Infertility Irregular menstruation, absence of menstruation, excessive bleeding Chronic lower backache
KD-6 Zhaohai 照海 Shining Sea 1 CUN inferior to the vertex of the MEDIAL MALLEOLUS, in a depression between the TENDONS of the TIBIALIS POSTERIOR and FLEXOR HALLUCIS LONGUS muscles. *OPENING POINT of the Yin Walker vessel*	Tonifies the Kidneys and clears deficiency heat Regulates the Yin Qiao mai (Yin Walker vessel) Calms the Mind Regulates the Lower Heater and Uterus	Dry throat and eyes of chronic nature (especially with the elderly), dizziness Constipation, hot skin diseases Night time epilepsy, Insomnia and somnolence Tightness of the inner aspect or muscles of the inner leg Anxiety, restlessness, sadness, fright and nightmares (spirit and will disharmony) Frequent urination, genital itching, Seminal emission Involuntary erection of the penis Oedema Absence of menstruation Irregular and painful menstruation Prolapse of uterus Difficult labour Red and white vaginal discharge (leucorrhoea)

Kidney Channel Points • Shen Jing Xue • 腎經穴

IDENTIFICATION	ACTION	INDICATIONS
KD-7 Fuliu 復溜 Returning Current In a depression on the sole when 2 CUN directly superior to KD-3 Taixi, in a depression, at the anterior border of the ACHILLES TENDON. *Jing-RIVER POINT* *METAL POINT of the Kidney channel*	Tonifies the Kidneys mainly Kidney Yang Resolves Dampness Lower Heater Regulates Sweating Strengthens the Lower Back Kidney Zone	Cold feeling in the body Aversion to cold Sore back, weak knees Oedema Impotence Scanty or abundant clear urine Lack of willpower Oedema of the legs Irregular menstruation Urinary dysfunction Under or oversweating response Lower back and kidney pain
KD-10 Yingu 陰谷 Yin Valley With the knee flexed, located at the medial end of the POPLITEAL crease, between the TENDONS of the SEMITENDINOSUS and SEMIMEMBRANOSUS muscles. *He-SEA POINT* *WATER POINT of the Kidney channel*	Clears Damp Heat from the Lower Heater Removes obstructions from the Channel	Abdominal pain and swelling, hernial disorders Frequent or painful urination Diarrhoea Vaginal discharge Genital pain and itching Impotence, conception difficulties Uterine bleeding Pain, stiffness and swelling of the inner aspect of the knee and thigh
KD-27 Shufu 俞府 Transport Mansion 2 CUN lateral to the midline or Ren mai (Controller vessel) in a depression on the lower border of the CLAVICLE.	Stimulates Kidney for reception of Qi Subdues ascending Qi	Asthma Bronchitis Chest pain Asthma Cough Anxiety and restlessness

Table 4.2 Functions of the Zang Fu (organ) and Zen Shiatsu (meridian) systems

ZANG FU 臟 腑	KIDNEY organ Shen zang 腎臟	BLADDER organ Pang Guang fu 膀胱腑
	Stores Essence (JING) Rules Reproduction and Growth Produces Marrow, fills Brain, controls Bones Foundation of Yin/Yang Governs Water Controls reception of Qi Opens into Ears Manifests in Head Hair Houses Willpower (Zhi)	Receives and excretes Urine
IMAGE	Strong and **Capable Ministers** from whom Technical Ability and Expertise are derived	**Governor** of the State Capital from where the Waters flows
GOVERNMENT	**DIRECTOR**	**REGIONAL MANAGER**

ZEN SHIATSU 神 指 土	KIDNEY meridian Shen jing 腎經	BLADDER meridian Pang Guang jing 膀胱經
	Governs Endocrine System (Glands and Hormones) Responds to Stress via Adrenal Glands Responds to Reproductive Drive via Sex Hormones Purifies the Blood Regulates Urine formation	Governs Autonomic Nervous System (ANS) Relates to Pituitary Gland and Kidney Hormonal System Controls Reproductive System and the Uterus Regulates elimination of Body Fluids and Urine via purification of Ki
BASIC	Controls Energy to Body for Instinctive Survival	Monitors and Purifies Energy for Instinctive Survival
SPECIFIC	**HORMONAL COMMUNICATION**	**NERVOUS COMMUNICATION**
GENERAL	**IMPETUS**	

Table 4.3 Zen Shiatsu correspondences: Bladder meridian

BLADDER meridian		Pang Guang jing 膀胱經
FACULTY	Spiritual Input	: ZHI via Kidney meridian
	Functions via	: Survival
	Represents	: Fluidity
	Supplemented by	: Nervous Communication
	Realised by	: Understanding
	Dominant Zone	: Back
	Embryological Layer	: Endoderm
	Meridian Nature	: Yang
	Tuning Time	: 3pm - 5pm
ANATOMY & PHYSIOLOGY	Medulla Oblongata	] Autonomic Nervous System
	Cerebellum	] (ANS)
	Spinal Cord	] Information, Movement, and
	Eyes	] Balance Response
	Hypothalamus	] Hormonal System
	Pituitary and Prostate Glands	] Reproductive System
	Uterus	]
	Kidneys	] Urinary System
	Ureters	] Fluid balance
	Bladder	]
PHYSICAL	ANS Disorders	Nasal Congestion
	Back & Neck Problems	Nervous Tension/Stress
	Chills - Back/Lower Body	Oedema
	Cramp	Palpitations
	Cystitis	Prostate Problems
	Distended Lower Hara	Retention of Urine
	Dizziness	Sciatica
	Eye/Vision Problems	Tight Shoulders
	Headaches	Urinary Disorders
	Incontinence	Uterine Problems
PSYCHOLOGICAL	Alertness	Overactive
	Anxiety	Oversensitive
	Complaining	Phobias
	Desire	Restful
	Easily Started	Seeking Balanced Lifestyle
	Evasive	Stress
	Fear	Sudden Tiredness
	Fretful	Suspicious Nature
	Issues of Character	Unnecessary Worry
	Neurotic	Weighing up the Situation

BLADDER meridian	Pang Guang jing 膀胱經

Table 4.4 Zen Shiatsu correspondences: Kidney meridian

KIDNEY meridian		Shen jing 腎經
FACULTY	Spiritual Input	: ZHI, Will
	Functions via	: Survival
	Represents	: Synchronisation
	Supplemented by	: Hormonal Communication
	Realised by	: Responding
	Dominant Zone	: Back
	Embryological Layer	: Endoderm
	Meridian Nature	: Yin
	Tuning Time	: 5pm - 7pm
ANATOMY & PHYSIOLOGY	Cerebrum	] Endocrine Gland System (EGS)
	Hypothalamus	] Hormonal System
	Pituitary Gland	] Information, Movement, and
	Ears	] Balance Response
	Adrenal and Prostate Glands	] Reproductive Response
	Kidneys	] Fluid Metabolism
	Ureters	] Urinary System
	Teeth	] Skeletal System
	Spine	]
	Bones	]
	Hair	] Integumentary System
PHYSICAL	Back Pain	Inflammation of Throat
	Baldness, Hair Loss	Lack of Body Tone
	Blood Problems	Oedema
	Coldness in Lower Body	Osteoporosis
	Darkness around Eyes	Poor Circulation
	Earache & Toothache	Premature Ageing
	Head Heaviness	Reproductive Problems
	Hearing Problems	Respiratory Disorders
	Hormonal Deficiency	Tension in Abdominal Muscles
	Impotence, Frigidity	Urinary Disorders, inc Stones
PSYCHOLOGICAL	Anxiety	Inability to Complete Things
	Apprehensive	Lack of Composure
	Continual Stress	Lack of Drive
	Easily Started	Listening Situations
	Easy Going	Overactiveness
	Excessive Fear	Phobias
	Exhaustion	Self Hate
	Feels Alone	Timidity
	Guilt	Timing
	How to Co-Ordinate	Working All the Time

Fig. 4.2 Anterior upper view: Zen Shiatsu Kidney and Bladder meridians

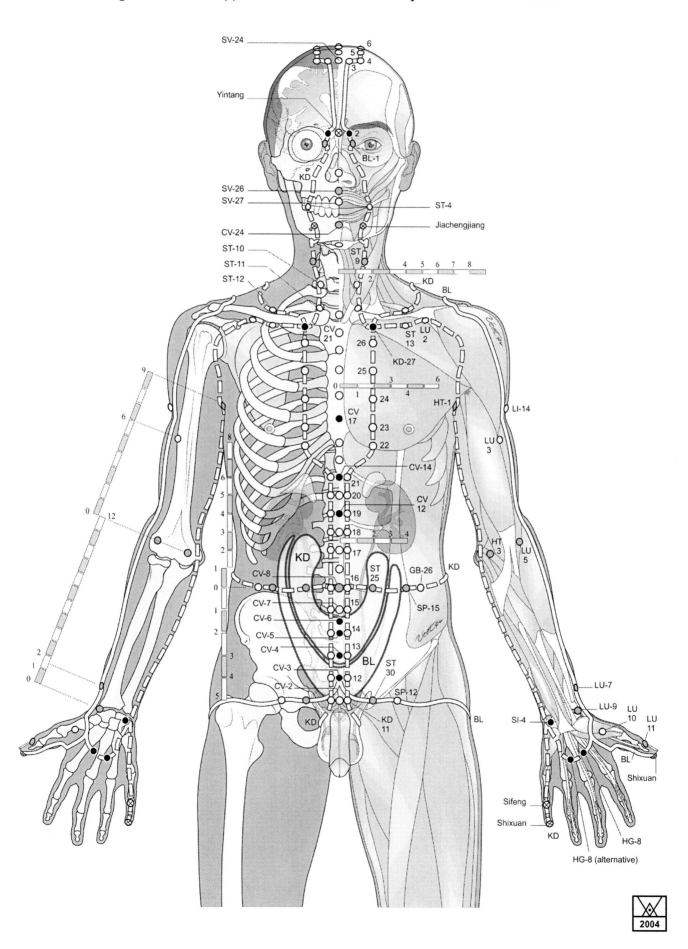

Fig. 4.3 Anterior lower view: Zen Shiatsu Kidney and Bladder meridians

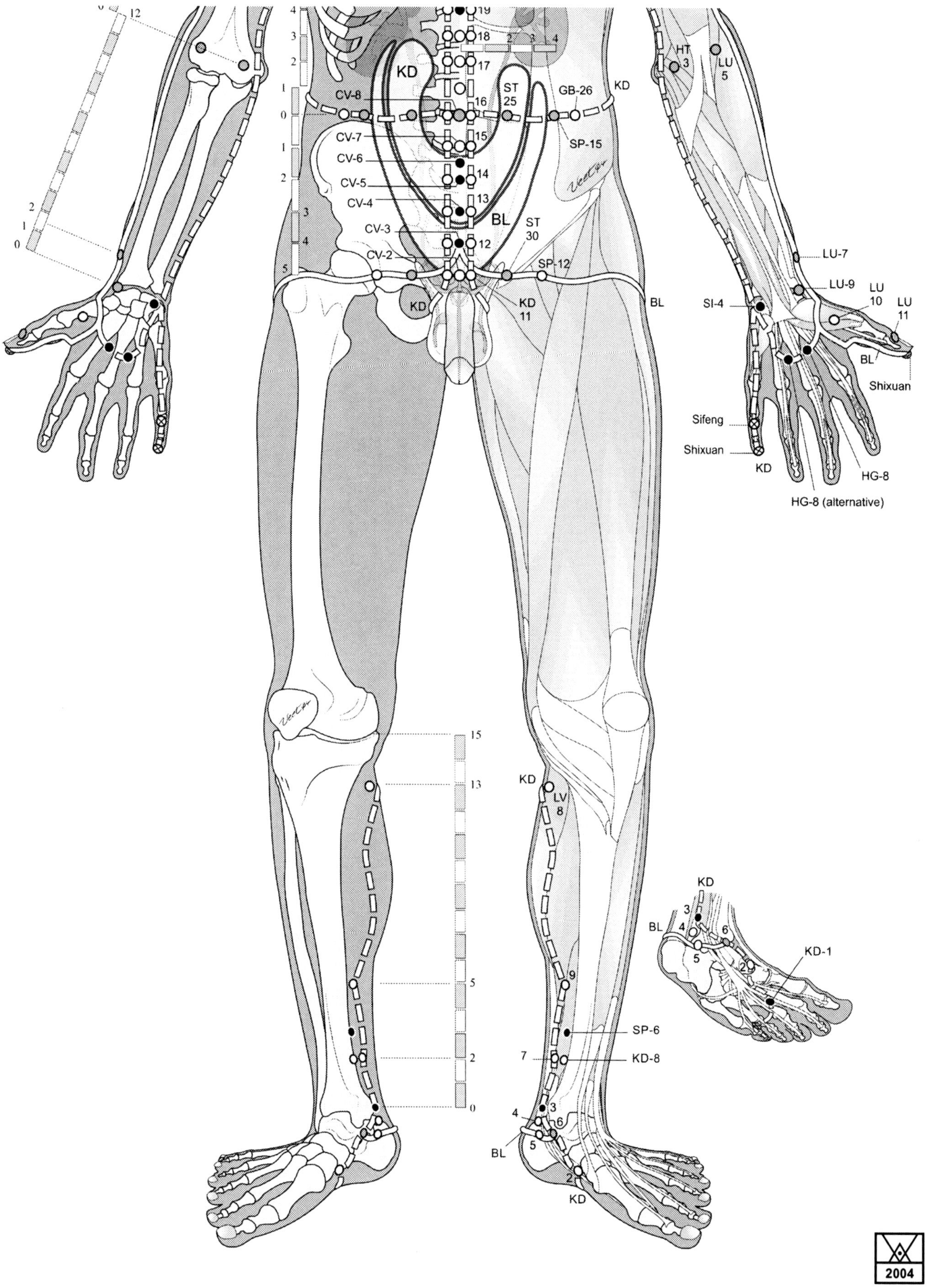

Fig. 4.4 Posterior upper view: Zen Shiatsu Kidney and Bladder meridians

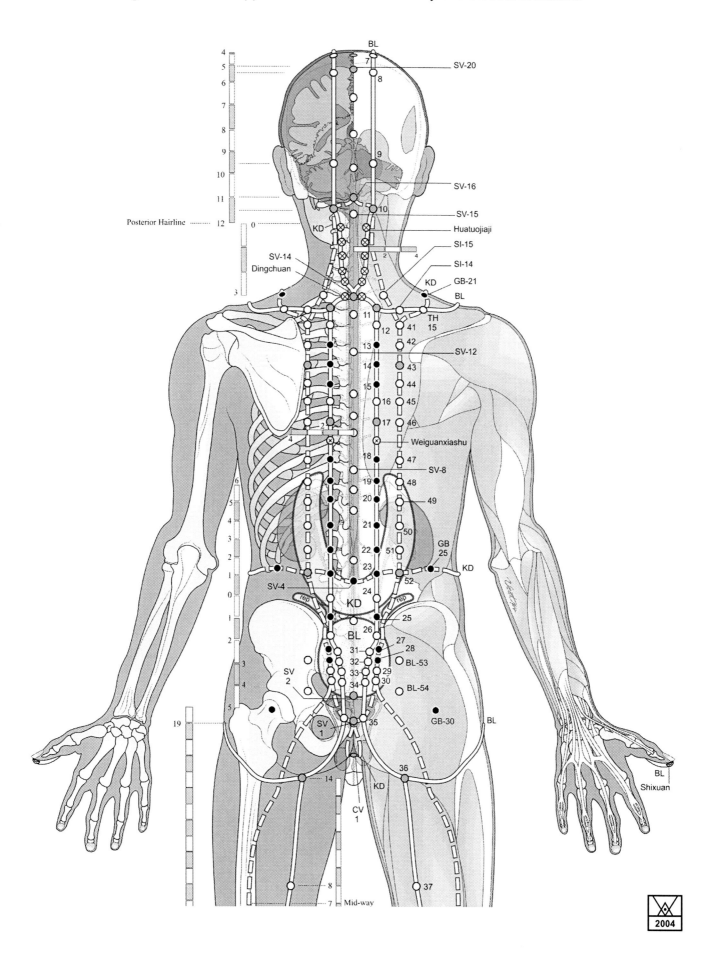

Fig. 4.5 Posterior lower view: Zen Shiatsu Kidney and Bladder meridians

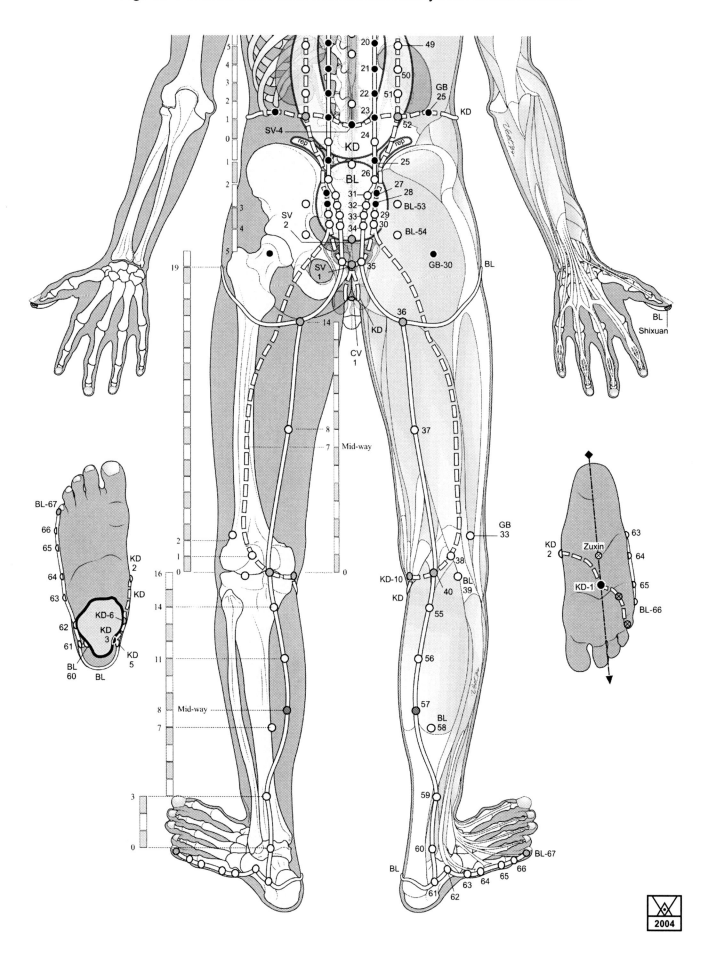

Fig. 4.6 Head cranial and lateral details: Zen Shiatsu Kidney and Bladder meridians

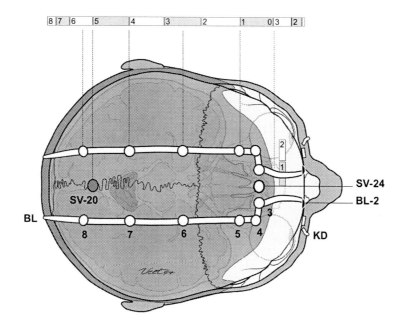

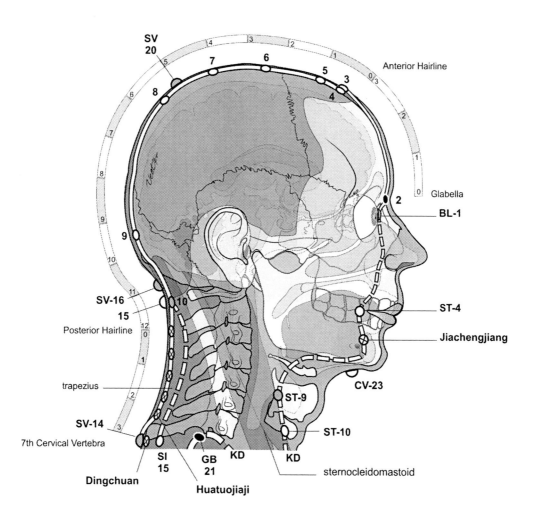

Fig. 4.7 Lower Arm and Hand details: Zen Shiatsu Kidney and Bladder meridians

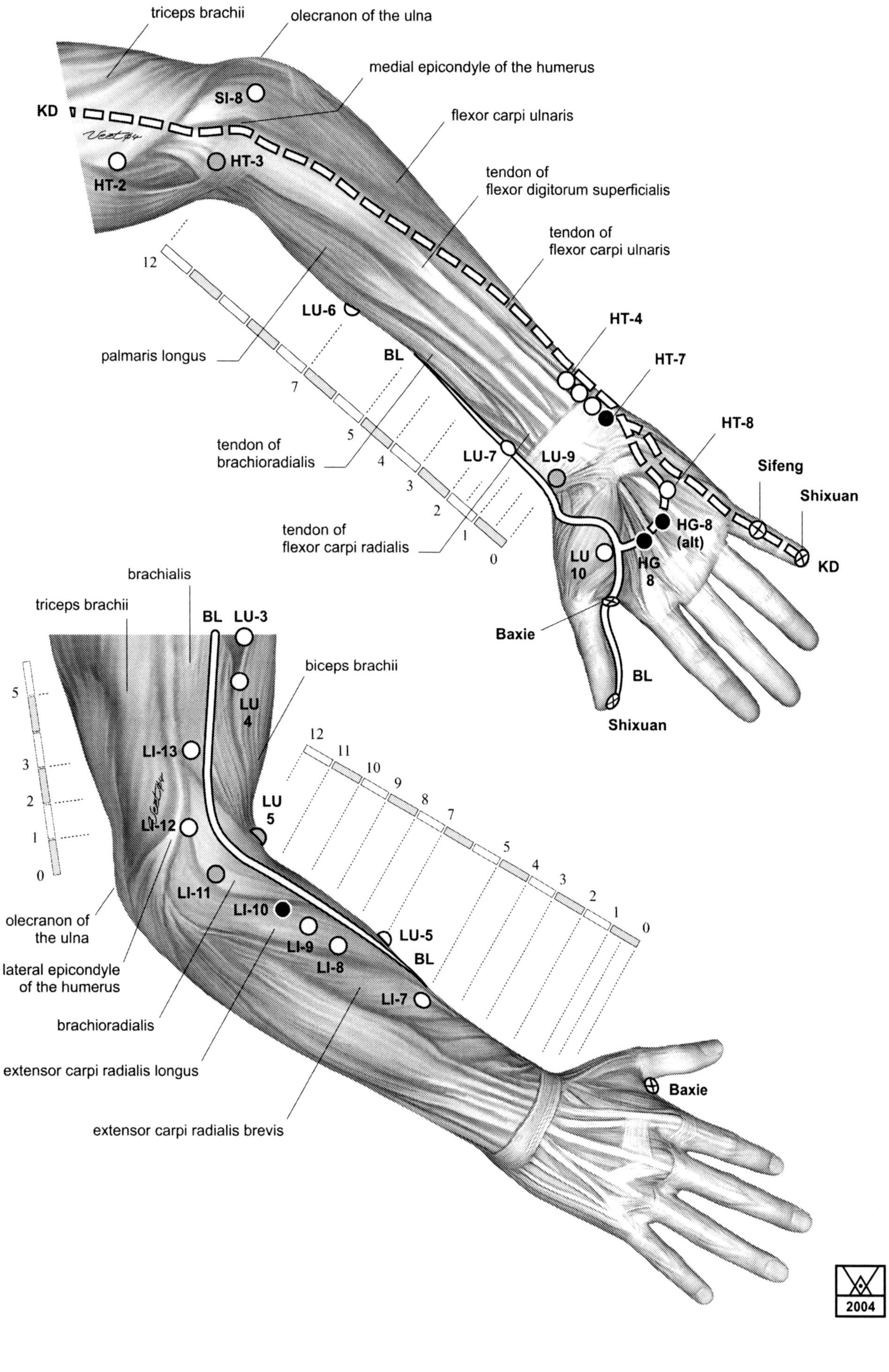

triceps brachii

olecranon of the ulna

medial epicondyle of the humerus

flexor carpi ulnaris

tendon of
flexor digitorum superficialis

tendon of
flexor carpi ulnaris

KD

SI-8

HT-3

HT-2

12

palmaris longus

LU-6

BL

7

tendon of
brachioradialis

5

4

LU-7

LU-9

HT-4

HT-7

HT-8

Sifeng

Shixuan

KD

3

2

tendon of
flexor carpi radialis

1

0

LU
10

HG
8

HG-8
(alt)

Baxie

BL

Shixuan

brachialis

triceps brachii

BL   LU-3

biceps brachii

5

3

LU
4

2

LI-13

1

0

LI-12

LU
5

12

11

10

9

8

7

5

4

3

2

1

0

LI-11

LI-10

LI-9

LI-8

LU-5

BL

olecranon of
the ulna

lateral epicondyle
of the humerus

brachioradialis

extensor carpi radialis longus

LI-7

Baxie

extensor carpi radialis brevis

2004

Fig. 4.8 Male Perineum details: Zen Shiatsu Kidney and Bladder meridians

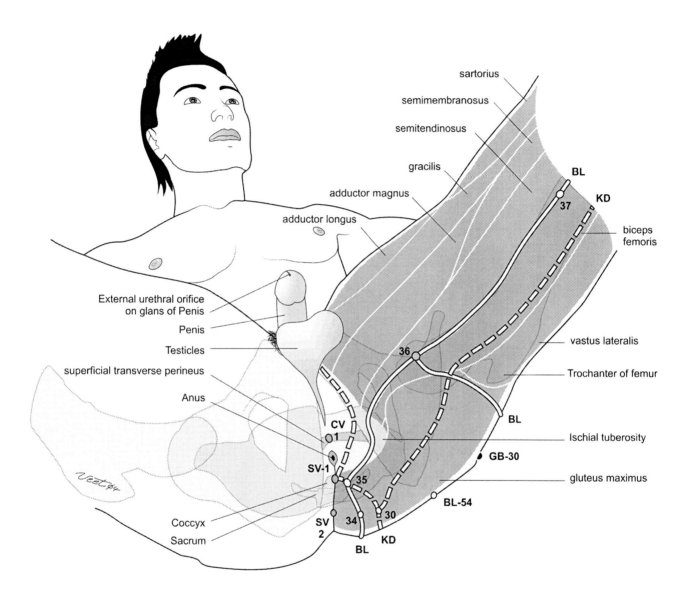

Fig. 4.9 Female Perineum details: Zen Shiatsu Kidney and Bladder meridians

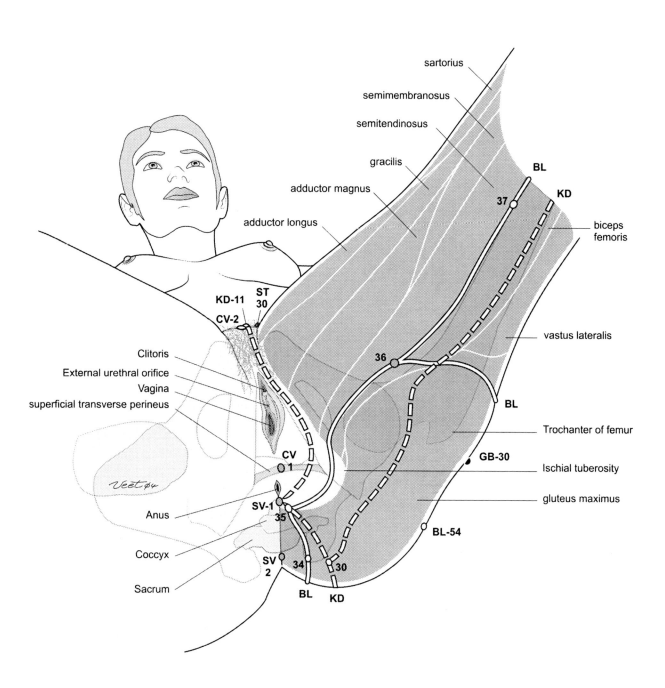

Fig. 4.10 Lower Leg and Foot details: Zen Shiatsu Kidney and Bladder meridians

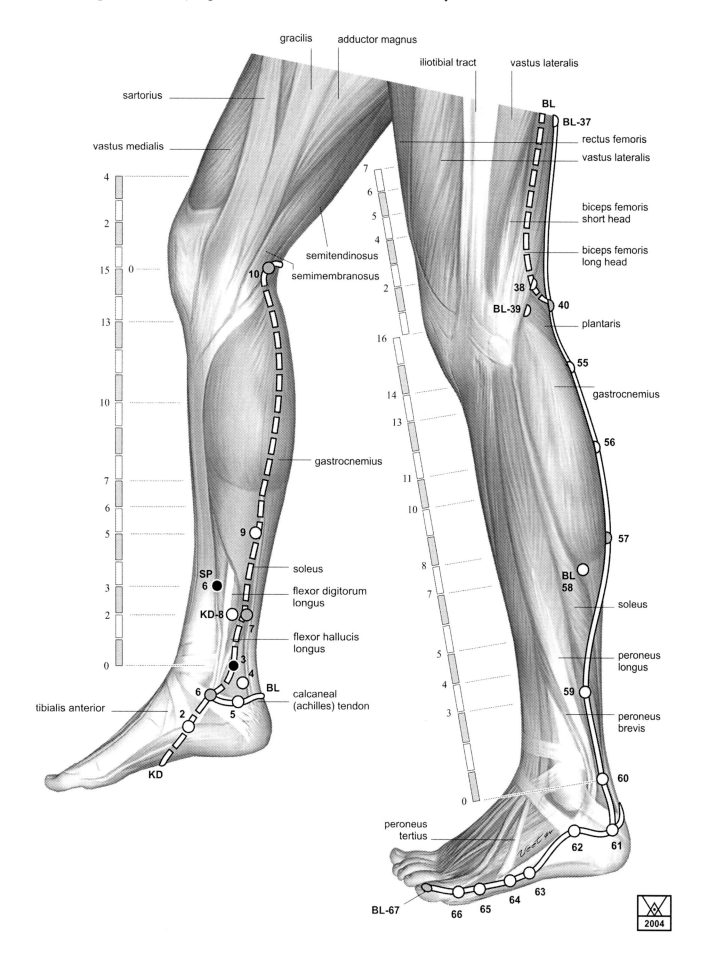

Fig. 4.11 Foot dorsal and plantar details: Zen Shiatsu Kidney and Bladder meridians

Foot: Dorsal view

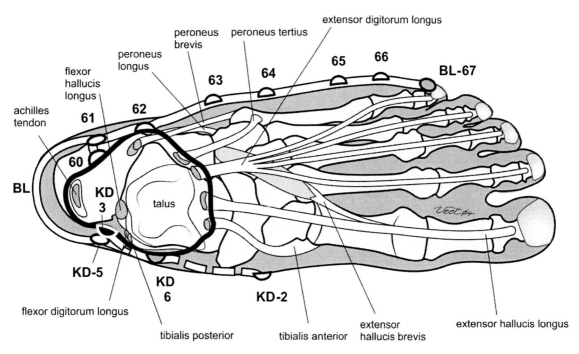

Foot: Plantar view

Chapter 5
the WOOD element

Gall Bladder
and
Liver

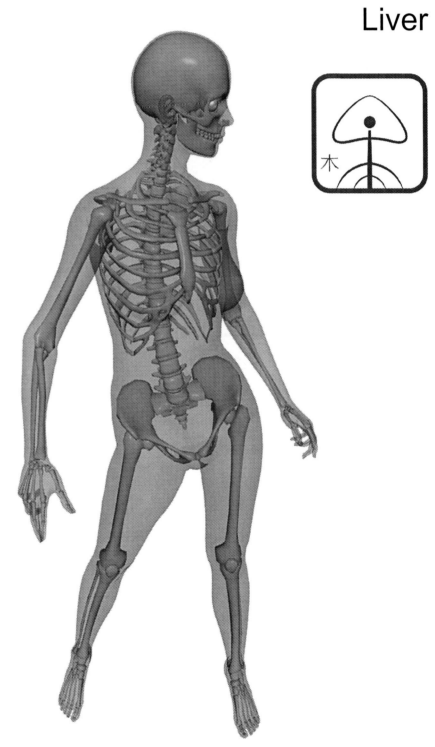

Fig. 5.1 The Five element sequences: WOOD

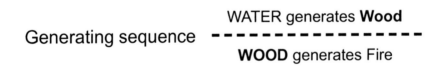

Generating sequence

WATER generates **Wood**

WOOD generates Fire

Control sequence

METAL controls **Wood**

WOOD controls Earth

Table 5.1 The Five element correspondences: WOOD

The WOOD element		Mu xing 木行
FACULTY	Spiritual	: Hun, Ethereal Soul Planning
	Celestial Stems	: Jia (stem 1) and Yi (stem 2)
	Earthly branches	: Yin (branch 3) and Mao (branch 4)
	Planet	: Jupiter
	Number	: 8
	Pentatonic note	: Jue, (Soh, 4th note of scale)
	Genetic aspiration	: Evolution via growth and adaptation
	Cycle	: Birth
	Yin/Yang	: Lesser Yang
	Quality	: Upward
ENVIRONMENTAL	Season	: Spring
	Phase of Moon	: Half moon increasing to full moon
	Climate	: Wind
	Direction	: East
	Colour	: Green
	Part of the Day	: Morning
BODY	Organ Yin	: Liver
	Yang	: Gall Bladder
	Tissue	: Tendons, Ligaments
	Skin Colour	: Green, Yellow
	Odour	: Rancid
	Branch	: Nails
	Sense Organ	: Eyes
	Senses	: Sight
	Fluid	: Tears
EMOTIONAL	Emotion	: Anger, Humour
	Sound, Voice	: Shouting, Clipped
	Action	: Twitching
FOOD (symbol)	Animal	: Chicken
	Taste	: Sour
	Fruit	: Plum
	Grain	: Wheat, Barley
	Vegetable	: Upward growth (celery, green peas, sprouts)

Gall Bladder Channel Points • Dan Jing Xue • 膽經穴

IDENTIFICATION	ACTION	INDICATIONS
GB-1 Tongziliao 瞳子髎 Pupil Bone-Hole 0.5 CUN lateral to the OUTER CANTHUS of the EYE, in the ORBITAL margin. *MEETING POINT of the Gall Bladder, Small Intestine and Triple Heater channels*	Clears Wind Heat Clears Fire Brightens the Eyes	Conjunctivitis Red, dry, painful eyes Migraine headaches Night/Colour blindness Dislike of light
GB-12 Wangu 完骨 Whole Bone In the depression immediately posterior and inferior to the MASTOID process *MEETING POINT of the Gall Bladder and Bladder channels*	Subdues Rising Qi Dispels Wind Exterior and Interior Calms the Mind	Posterior migraine headaches on the Gall Bladder channel Earache and toothache Epilepsy Inflammation of the Middle Ear Insomnia, throat pain and stiff neck due to emotional crisis
GB-14 Yangbai 陽白 Yang White On the forehead, superior to the PUPIL, located 1 CUN above the middle of the Eyebrow. *MEETING POINT of the Gall Bladder, Triple Heater, Stomach, and Large Intestine channels and the Yang Tie vessel*	Dispels Exterior Wind Benefits Head and Eyes	Facial paralysis Frontal headache Dizziness, Pain over the eyebrows. Eye pain, blurred vision, night blindness Tears on exposure to the wind Itching of the eyelids, pupil or mouth Drooping of the eyelid Deviation of the mouth
GB-20 Fengchi 風池 Wind Pool In the hollow between the OCCIPITAL PROTRUBERANCE and the MASTOID bone, level with SV-16 Fengfu and between the upper STERNO-CLEIDO-MASTOID muscle and TRAPEZIUS muscle. *MEETING POINT of the Gall Bladder and Triple Heater channels, Yang Walker vessel and the Yang Tie vessel*	Dispels Wind: Exterior and Interior Subdues Liver Yang / Fire Calms the Mind Clears the Brain Sea of Marrow	Exterior: Pronounced headache, stiff neck, shoulder and back pain Interior: Vertigo, dizziness Occipital headaches Eye and Ear problems Insomnia, dizziness, vertigo Poor memory Hypertension

Gall Bladder Channel Points • Dan Jing Xue • 膽經穴

IDENTIFICATION	ACTION	INDICATIONS
GB-21 Jianjing 肩井 Shoulder Well At the highest point of the SHOULDER, halfway between SV-14 Dazhui and the ACROMION, at the TRAPEZIUS muscle. *MEETING POINT of the Gall Bladder, Triple Heater and Stomach channels with the Yang Tie vessel* **** Contra-indicated in pregnancy ****	Relaxes Tendons including Ligaments Re-directs Qi downward Promotes Delivery Facilitates Lactation	Tender and painful neck and shoulders Cough, hiccup, difficulty inhaling, Asthma Digestive problems Retention of placenta Post Partum haemorrhage Difficult labour Insufficient lactation Mastitis
GB-24 Riyue 日月 Sun and Moon Directly below the NIPPLE in the 7th INTERCOSTAL SPACE (between the 7th and 8th RIBS). *FRONT Mu-COLLECTING POINT of the Gall Bladder* *MEETING POINT of the Gall Bladder and Spleen channels with the Yang Tie vessel*	Damp Heat cleared from Liver and Gall Bladder Promotes Liver and Gall Bladder function Spreads Liver Qi	Jaundice Hypochondriac pain Heavy feeling in Middle Heater Nausea, sticky yellow tongue coating Gallstones Hypochondriac pain and distension Tight chest, depression Indecision
GB-25 Jingmen 京門 Capital Gate At the tip of the free end of the 12th RIB. *FRONT Mu-COLLECTING POINT of the Liver*	Tonifies Kidneys Yin or Yang aspects Resolves Dampness Lower Heater Expels stones	Breathing problems Painful urinary dysfunction Restless foetal disorder Oedema Hypochondriac, abdominal or lower back pain Inflammation of Kidney Urinary tract stones
GB-30 Huantiao 環跳 Jumping Circle One third the distance from the prominence of the GREATER TROCHANTER of the FEMUR to the SACRAL-COCCYGEAL HIATUS. *MEETING POINT of the Gall Bladder and Bladder channels*	Tonifies Qi and Blood Removes obstructions from Channel Resolves Damp Heat Lower Heater	Whole body tiredness with stagnant feeling Hip joint and leg pain Sciatica Rheumatism Itchy anus or groin Vaginal discharge Urethritis Lower back or groin pain

Gall Bladder Channel Points • Dan Jing Xue • 膽經穴

IDENTIFICATION	ACTION	INDICATIONS
GB-34 Yanglingquan 楊陵泉 Yang Mound Spring In the hollow, anterior and inferior to the head of the FIBULA, below the lateral aspect of the KNEE. *He-SEA POINT* *EARTH POINT of the Gall bladder channel* *Hui-MEETING POINT of sinews, tendons and ligaments* *Ma Dan-yang HEAVENLY STAR POINT*	Smooths Liver Qi Subdues rebellious Qi Resolves Damp Heat Relaxes Tendons including Ligaments	Hypochondriac pain Gallstones Nausea and vomiting Hepatitis Knee pain, Oedema Sciatica Rheumatism Muscular atrophy Cramps and spasms *Woody* like tight musculature
GB-40 Qiuxu 丘墟 Mound of Ruins Anterior and inferior to the LATERAL MALLEOLUS, in the hollow on the lateral side of the TENDON of the EXTENSOR DIGITORUM LONGUS muscle. *Yuan-SOURCE POINT*	Smooths Liver Qi, harmonises Liver and Gall Bladder Removes obstructions from Channel	Gallstones Hypochondriac pain Distension with sighing Indecision Pain in neck, side, hip, knee and ankle Weak joints with swelling inc. foot
GB-44 Zuqiaoyin 足竅陰 Foot Portals of Yin About 0.1 CUN from the lateral corner of the 4th TOENAIL, level with the base line of the nail. *Jing-WELL POINT* *METAL POINT of the Gall bladder channel*	Subdues Liver Yang Soothes Eyes Calms the Mind	Migraine headaches Obstruction of throat Red, painful eyes Insomnia Agitation

Liver Channel Points • Gan Jing Xue • 肝經穴

IDENTIFICATION	ACTION	INDICATIONS
LV-1 Dadun 大敦 Big Sincerity 0.1 CUN lateral to the corner of the big TOENAIL, level with the base of the nail. *Jing-WELL POINT* *WOOD POINT of the Liver channel*	Resolves Damp Heat Lower Heater zone Contains the Blood Spreads Liver Qi	Genital itching, swelling and pain Urinary infection and incontinence Uterine bleeding or blood in urine or stool Irregular menstruation Distension of hypogastrium Urinary pain
LV-3 Taichong 太衝 Supreme Thoroughfare At the dorsal junction between the 1st and 2nd METATARSAL BONES, in the hollow 2 CUN proximal to the margin of the web. *Yuan-SOURCE POINT* *Shu-STREAM POINT* *EARTH POINT of the Liver channel* *Ma Dan-yang HEAVENLY STAR POINT*	Subdues Liver Yang Calms the Mind Smooths Liver Qi Expels Interior Wind	Migraines, headaches with dizziness Rebellious Qi Stress, irritability and frustration Repressed anger Premenstrual tension Irregular menstruation Calms spasms and cramping of the muscles
LV-4 Zhongfeng 中封 Middle Seal Anterior to the vertex of the medial MALLEOLUS, in the hollow medial to the TENDON of the TIBIALIS ANTERIOR muscle. *Jing-RIVER POINT* *METAL POINT of the Liver channel*	Smooths Liver Qi Lower Heater zone Painful obstruction syndrome	Hernial disorders Distension of hypogastrium due to stagnant Liver Qi Urinary retention Impotence Pain and swelling of the ankle
LV-5 Ligou 蠡溝 Woodworm Canal 5 CUN superior to the vertex of the medial MALLEOLUS on the medial posterior border of the TIBIA. *Luo-CONNECTING POINT*	Promotes the smooth flow of Liver Qi Resolves Damp Heat Regulates Menstruation Alleviates Plumstone Qi (globus hystericus)	Distension of hypogastrium Sexual dysfunction : impotence, seminal emission, incessant erection of penis Pain preceediing urination, retention of urine Lower back pain and spasm Vaginal discharge Cloudy urine Painful menses, irregular menstruation Utero-vaginal prolapse Throat tension due to emotional stress Fear, fright, depression, belching and frequent swallowing

Liver Channel Points • Gan Jing Xue • 肝經穴

IDENTIFICATION	ACTION	INDICATIONS
LV-8 Ququan 曲泉 Spring at the Crook With the KNEE flexed, in the depression at the medial end of the POPLITEAL crease, between the upper border of the medial EPICONDYLE of the FEMUR and the TENDON of the SEMI MEMBRANOSUS muscle. *He-SEA POINT* *WATER POINT of the Liver channel*	Resolves Dampness Hot or Cold Lower Heater zone Nourishes Blood Relaxes Tendons	Urinary retention Cloudy urine Burning urination Vaginal discharge Genital itching Irregular menstruation Impotence Arthritic pain Stiffness and/or swelling at the medial aspect of the thigh
LV-13 Zhangmen 章門 Completion Gate At the anterior and inferior free end of the 11th RIB. *FRONT Mu-COLLECTING POINT of the Spleen* *Hui-MEETING POINT of the five Zang (Lung, Heart, Liver, Spleen and Kidneys)* *MEETING POINT of the Liver and Gall Bladder channels*	Smooths Liver Qi Relieves retention of food	Liver / Spleen disharmony Spleen Qi not ascending Loose stools Abdominal distension Stomach Qi not descending Retention of food Belching Epigastric fullness
LV-14 Qimen 期門 Cyclic Gate On the MAMILLARY line directly below the NIPPLE in the 6th INTERCOSTAL SPACE (between the 6th and 7th RIBS), 4 CUN lateral to the midline. *FRONT Mu-COLLECTING POINT of the Liver*	Smooths Liver Qi Cools the Blood	Liver / Stomach disharmony Stomach Qi not descending Belching Nausea, vomiting Hypochondriac pain and distension Depression Full and tight constricted chest Difficult breathing Liver fog (can't plan) Skin rashes Inflammation of the Gall Bladder and the Pancreas

Table 5.2 Functions of the Zang Fu (organ) and Zen Shiatsu (meridian) systems

ZANG FU 臟腑	LIVER organ Gan zang 肝臟	GALL BLADDER organ Dan fu 膽腑
	Ensures the smooth flow of Qi Stores the Blood Controls the Sinews (Tendons and Ligaments) Opens into the Eyes Manifests in the Nails Houses the Ethereal Soul (HUN)	Stores and excretes Bile Controls Judgement Controls the Sinews (Tendons and Ligaments)
IMAGE	Like an **Army General** who plans the Overall Strategy	The impartial **Officer** who makes Decisions
GOVERNMENT	**GENERAL**	**LIEUTENANT**

ZEN SHIATSU 神指士	LIVER meridian Gan jing 肝經	GALL BLADDER meridian Dan jing 膽經
	Stores the Nutrients and vital Energy Plans the distribution of Energy Stores and detoxifies Blood Cultivates resistance against Disease	Distribution of Nutrients to Body Balances Energy through Hormones, Bile secretion, Gastric Acid and Insulin Responds to Liver's Plans by deciding Course of Action
BASIC	Detoxification, Planning and Storage of Ki	Delivers Nutrients for Maintainance
SPECIFIC	**PLANNING**	**DECISION MAKING**
GENERAL	**DISTRIBUTION OF KI**	

Table 5.3 Zen Shiatsu correspondences: Gall Bladder meridian

GALL BLADDER meridian		Dan jing 膽經
FACULTY	Spiritual Input	: HUN via Liver meridian
	Functions via	: Etheric Body
	Represents	: Accomplishment
	Supplemented by	: Decision Making
	Realised by	: Resolving
	Dominant Zone	: Side
	Embryological Layer	: Mesoderm
	Meridian Nature	: Yang
	Tuning Time	: 11pm - 1am
ANATOMY & PHYSIOLOGY	Thyroid	] Hormonal System (EGS)
	Parathyroids	]
	Gall Bladder	] Digestive System
	Pancreas	
	Female, Male Genitalia	] Reproductive System
	Ova	] Sexual Vitality
	Spermatozoa	]
	Eyes	] Co-ordination
	Joints, Ligaments	] Musco-Skeletal System
	Tendons	]
PHYSICAL	Abdominal Distension	Lack of Sexual Response
	Biliary Pain/Gallstones	Lack of Sexual Vigour
	Bitter Taste	Jaundice, Yellow Eyes
	Blurred Vision	Joint Pain, Stiffness
	Diarrhoea	Migraine Headaches
	Difficulty Twisting	Nutritional Disorders
	Eye Problems	Pain in Flanks, Genitals
	Fatigue	Poor Digestion of Fats
	Infertility	Pyrosis (Heartburn)
	Intercostal Neuralgia	Shoulder Tension
PSYCHOLOGICAL	Agitated During Sleep	Indecisive
	Anger - Rage	Issues of Choice
	At Wits' End	Officious
	Disappointed	Overbearing
	Discriminate	Overcompetitive
	Easily Upset	Overconcentrative
	Fast Food/Life Freak	Resentment
	High Achiever	Responsibility
	Impatient	Stuckness
	Inability to Act	Tiredness after Stress

GALL BLADDER meridian   Dan jing 膽經

Table 5.4 Zen Shiatsu correspondences: Liver meridian

LIVER meridian			Ganjing 肝經
FACULTY	Spiritual Input	:	HUN, Ethereal Soul
	Functions via	:	Etheric Body
	Represents	:	Flow of Ki
	Supplemented by	:	Planning
	Realised by	:	Aspiring
	Dominant Zone	:	Side
	Embryological Layer	:	Mesoderm
	Meridian Nature	:	Yin
	Tuning Time	:	1am - 3am
ANATOMY & PHYSIOLOGY	Liver	]	Digestive System/Nutrional
		]	Blood Quality
	Female, Male Genitalia	]	Hormonal System (EGS)
	Fertilized Egg (Zygote)	]	Reproductive System
		]	Sexual Vitality
		]	Reproduction/Early Development
	Eyes	]	Co-ordination
	Joints, Ligaments	]	Musco-Skeletal System
	Tendons	]	
	Nails	]	Integumentary System
PHYSICAL	Alcohol Poisoning		Joint Pain, Stiffness
	Cracked Nails		Lack of Sexual Energy
	Dizziness		Liver Problems
	Eye, Visual Disorders		Migraine Headaches
	Fevers		Nausea
	Flatulence		Poor Digestion (Fats)
	Haemorrhoids		Sexual Organ Dysfunctions
	Hypochondriac Pain		Sluggish due to Toxins
	Infertility		Tension in Flanks
	Jaundice		Weight Loss
PSYCHOLOGICAL	Anger		Opinionated
	Bad Tempered		Overdemanding
	Depression		Overindulgence
	Disappointment		Perseverance
	Easily Disturbed		Psycho-sexual Endurance
	Emotionally Sensitive		Repressed Emotions
	Irritable		Resentment
	Lack of Patience		Sudden Inspiration
	Loud Mouthed		Tunnel Vision
	Observer		Worry over Future

Fig. 5.2 Anterior upper view: Zen Shiatsu Gall Bladder and Liver meridians

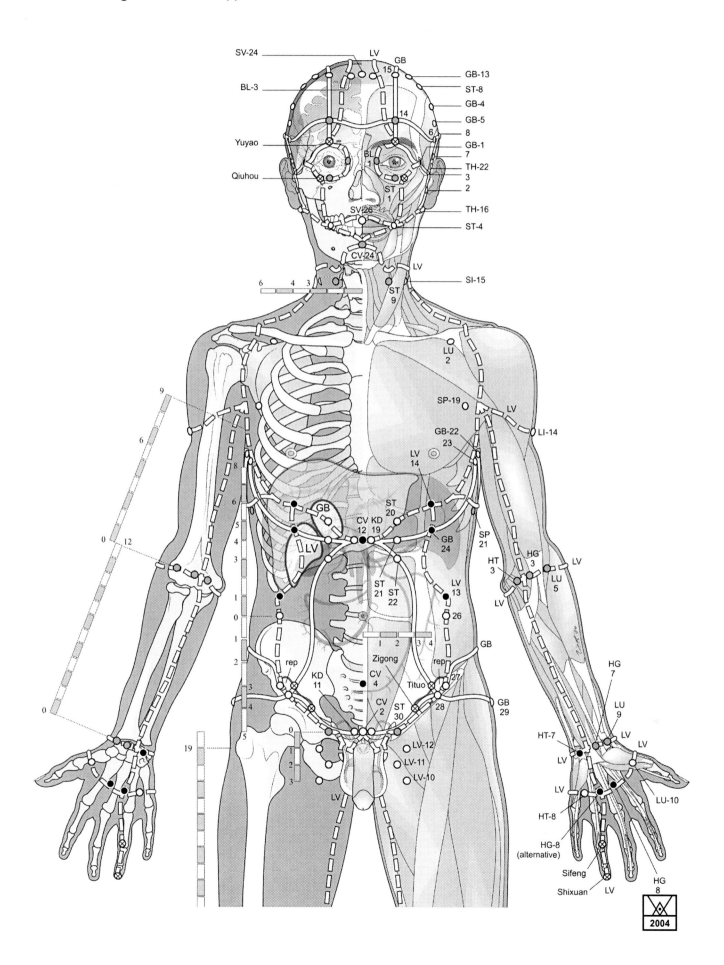

Fig. 5.3 Anterior lower view: Zen Shiatsu Gall Bladder and Liver meridians

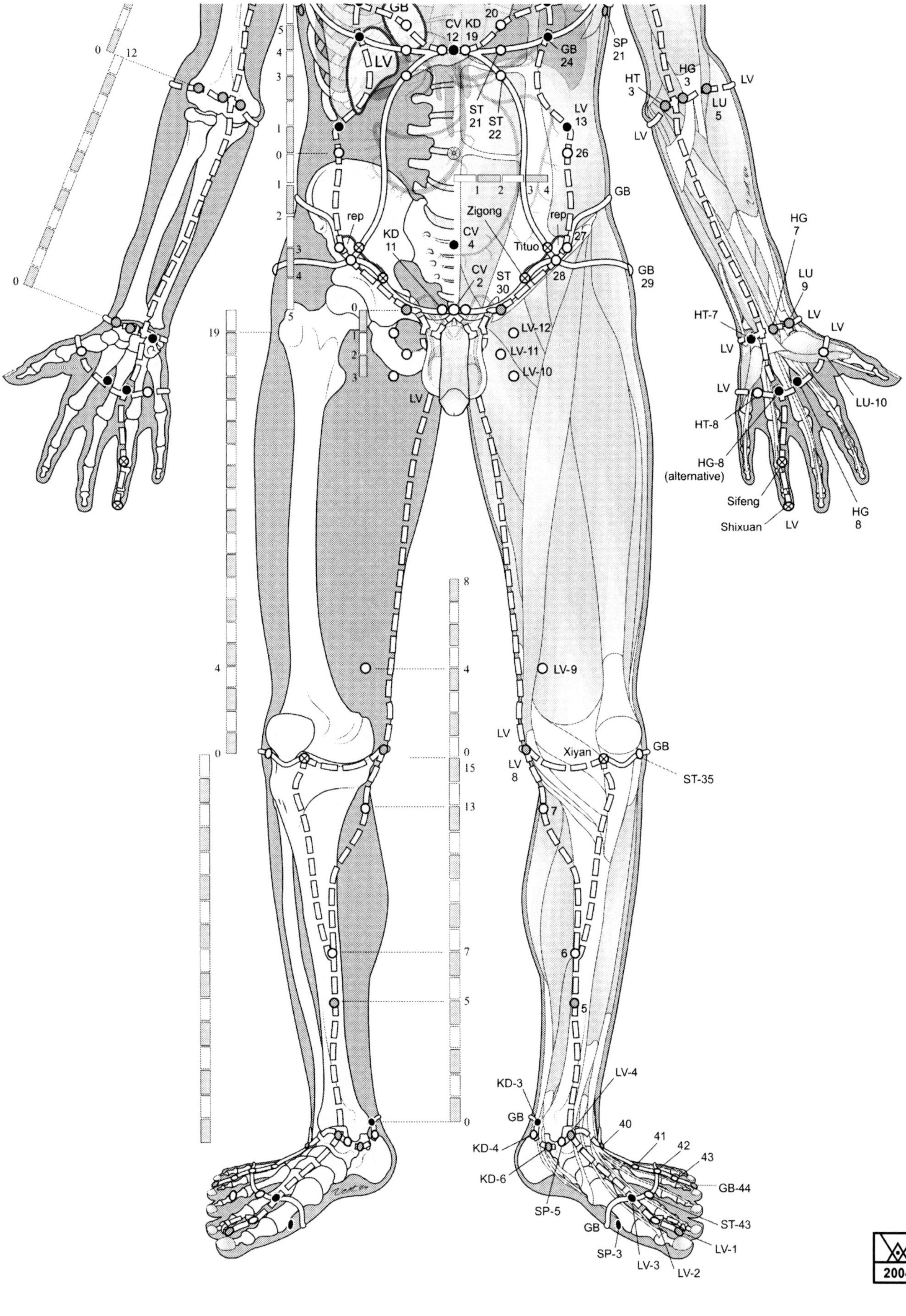

2004

Fig. 5.4 Posterior upper view: Zen Shiatsu Gall Bladder and Liver meridians

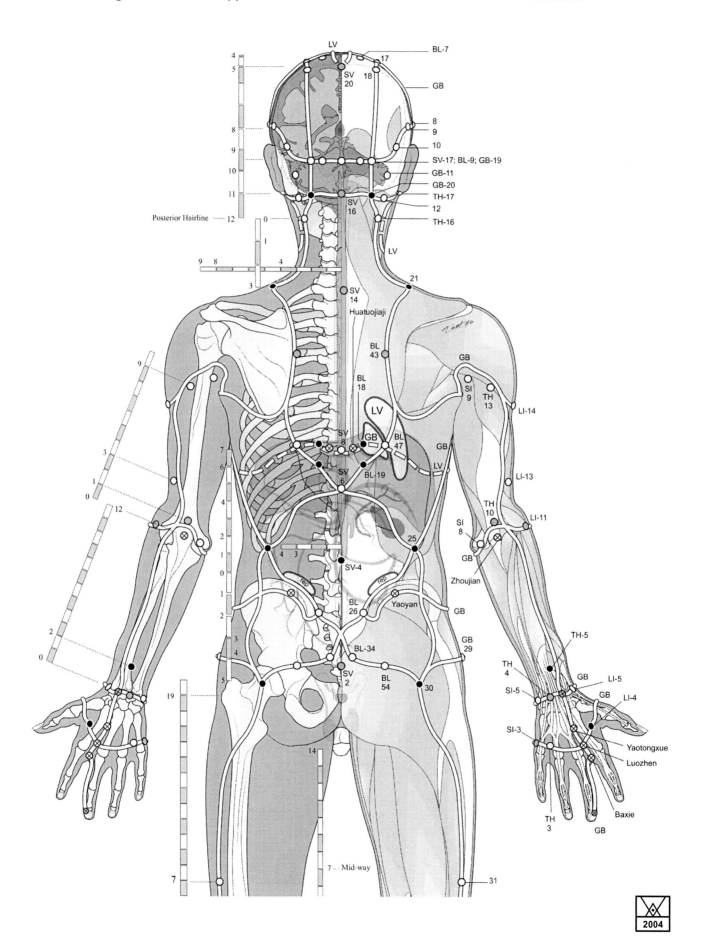

Fig. 5.5 Posterior lower view: Zen Shiatsu Gall Bladder and Liver meridians

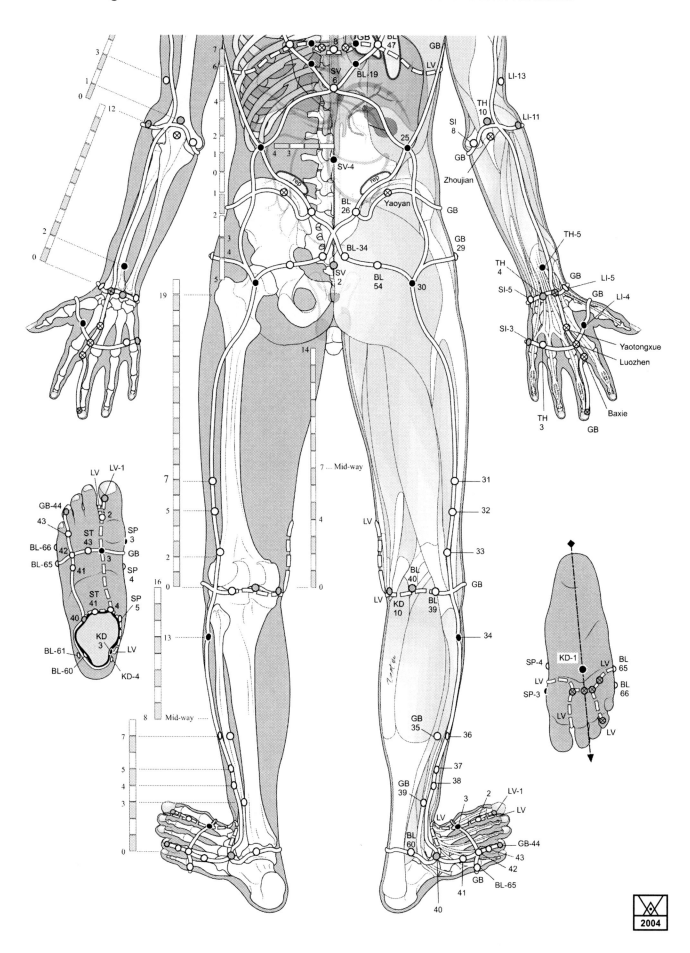

Fig. 5.6 Posterior-lateral upper view: Zen Shiatsu Gall Bladder and Liver meridians

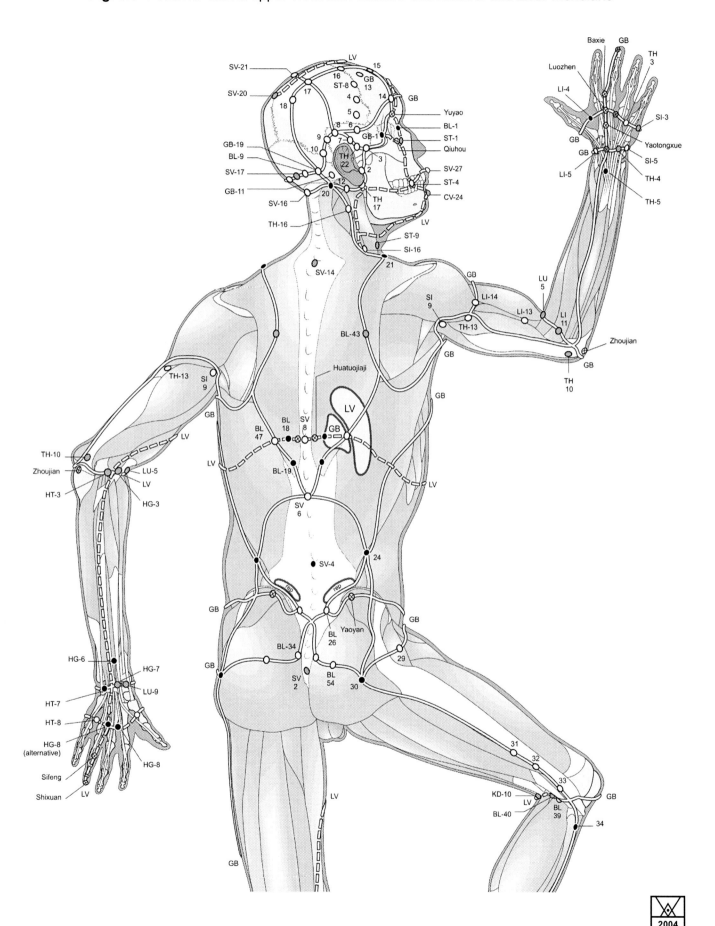

Fig. 5.7 Posterior-lateral upper view: Zen Shiatsu Gall Bladder and Liver meridians

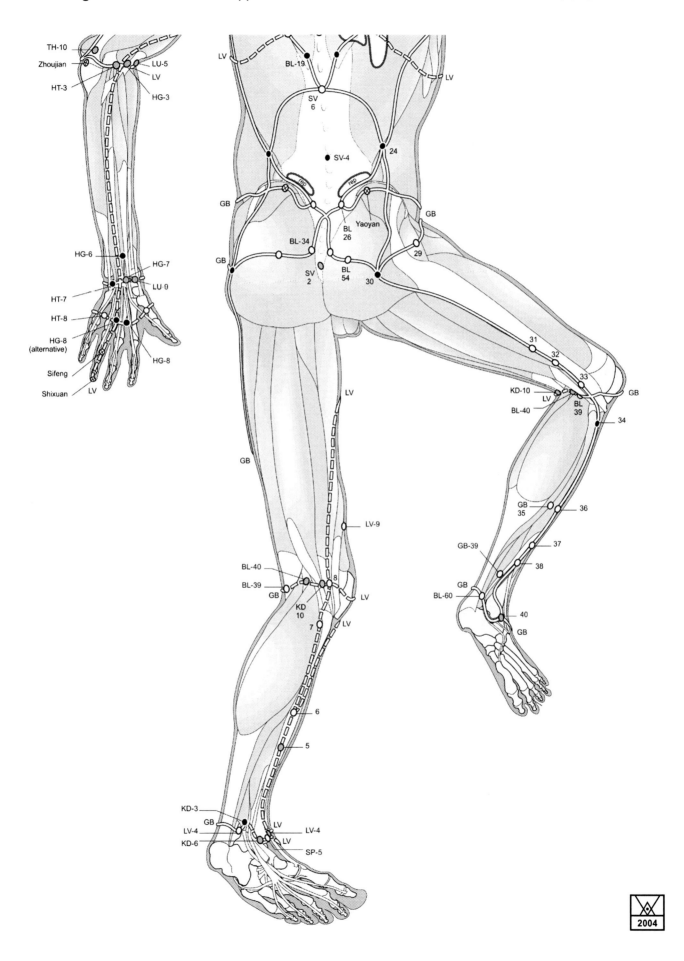

Fig. 5.8 Head cranial and lateral details: Zen Shiatsu Gall Bladder and Liver meridians

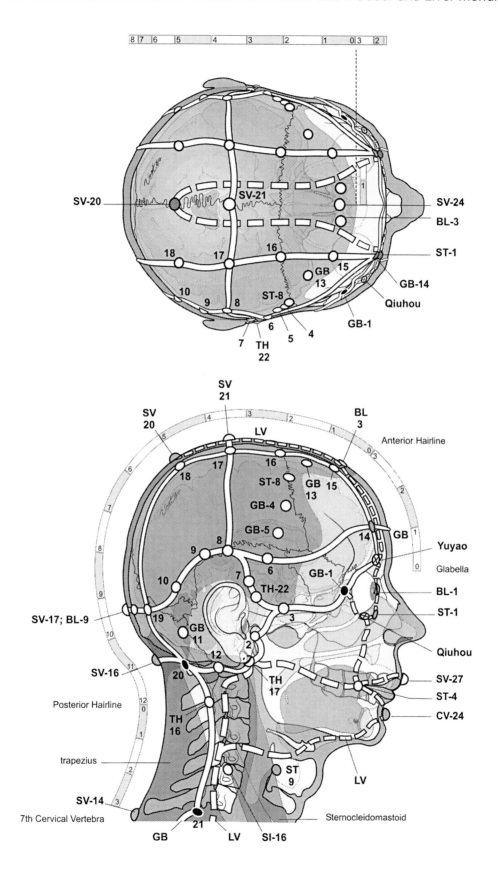

Fig. 5.9 Lower Arm and Hand details: Zen Shiatsu Gall Bladder and Liver meridians

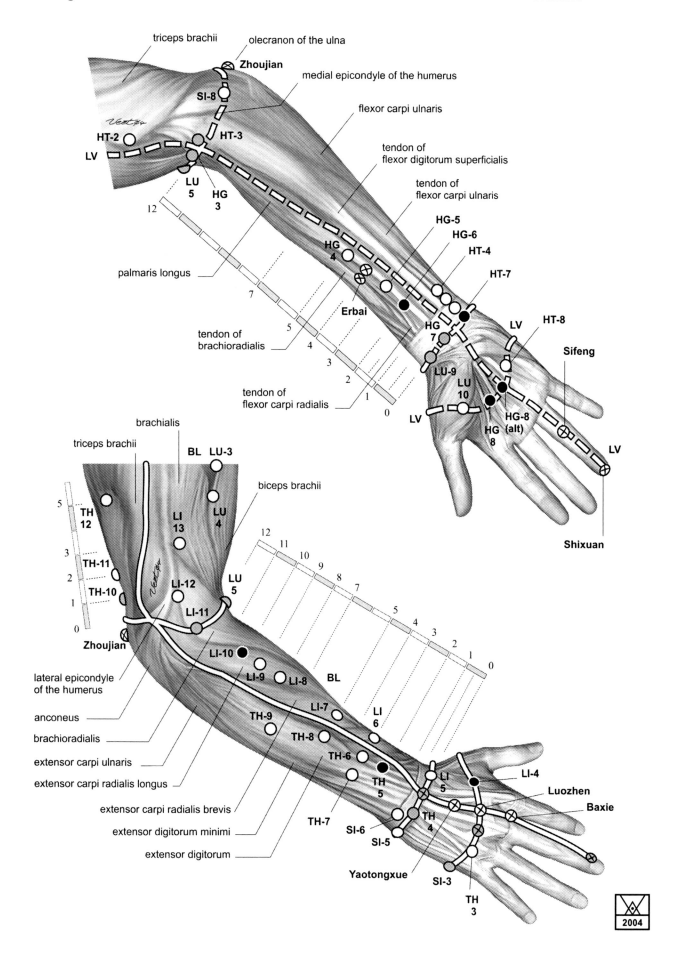

Fig. 5.10 Male Perineum details: Zen Shiatsu Gall Bladder and Liver meridians

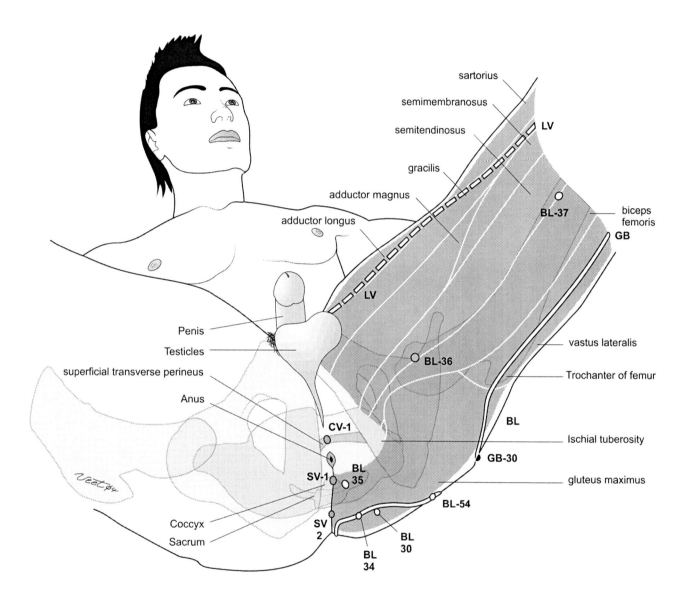

Fig. 5.11 Female Perineum details: Zen Shiatsu Gall Bladder and Liver meridians

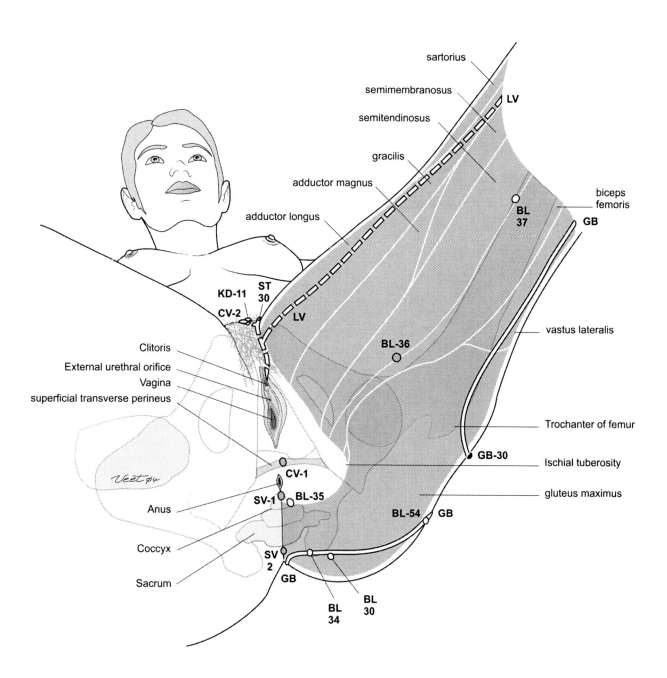

Fig. 5.12 Lower Leg and Foot details: Zen Shiatsu Gall Bladder and Liver meridians

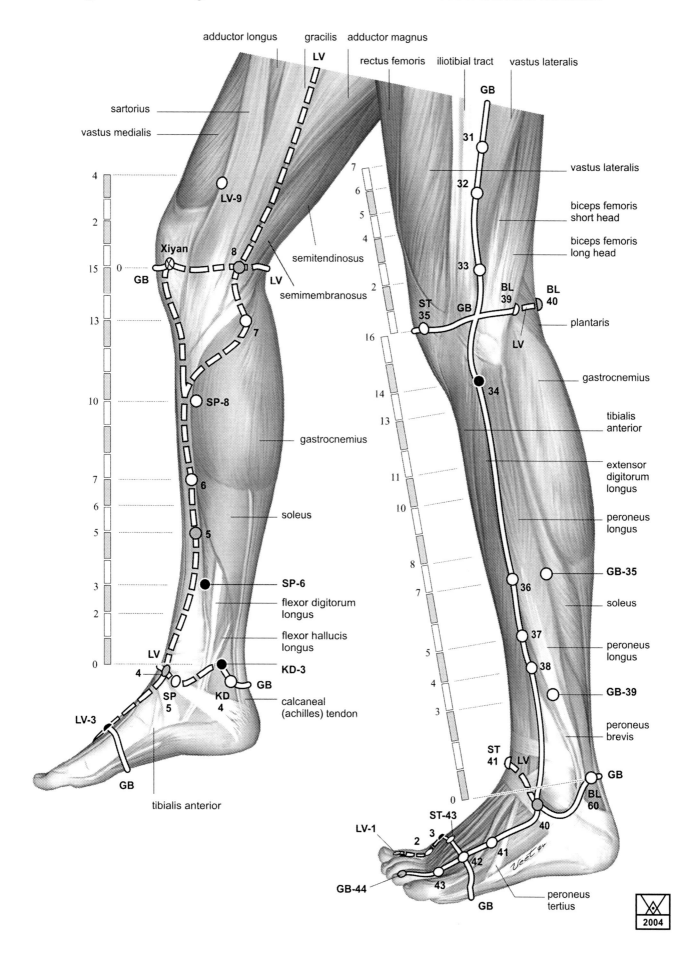

Fig. 5.13 Foot dorsal and plantar details: Zen Shiatsu Gall Bladder and Liver meridians

Foot: Dorsal view

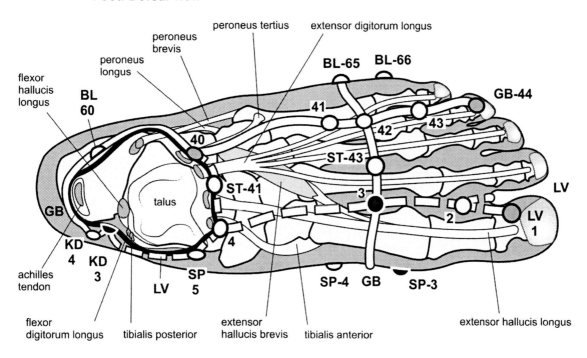

Foot: Plantar view

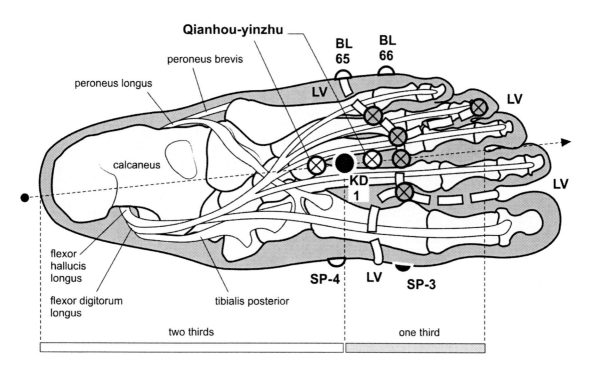

Chapter 6
the FIRE element part one

Heart
and
Small Intestine

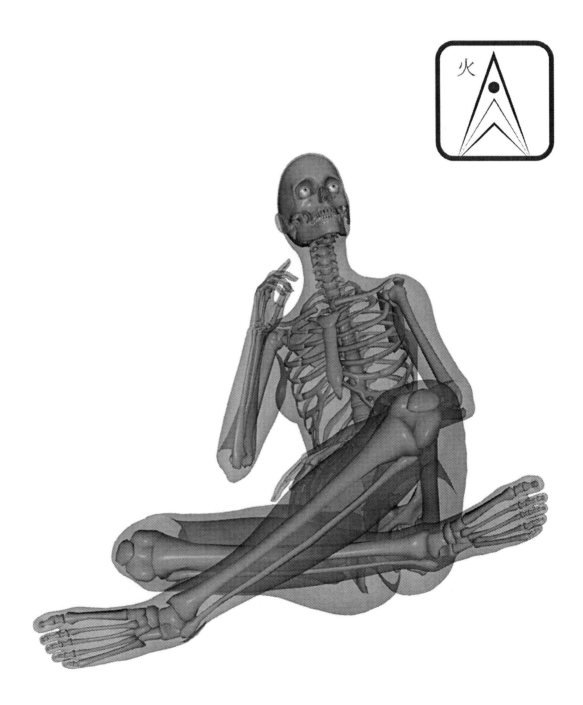

Fig. 6.1 The Five element sequences: FIRE

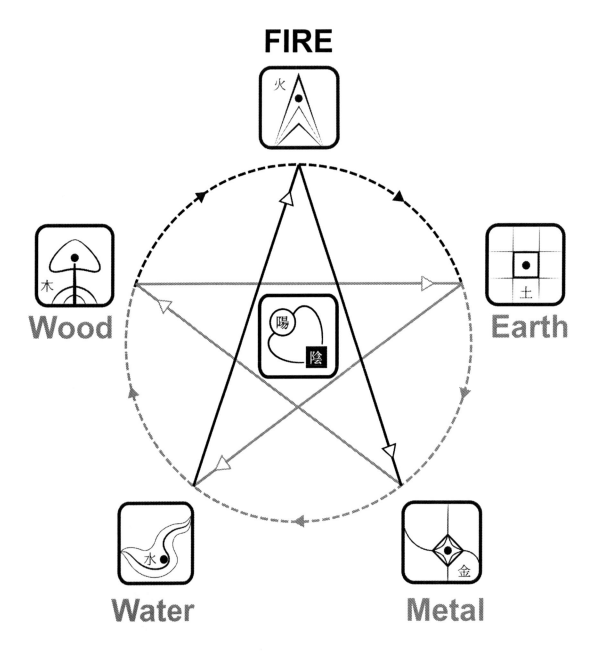

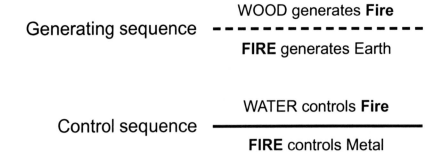

Generating sequence — WOOD generates **Fire** / **FIRE** generates Earth

Control sequence — WATER controls **Fire** / **FIRE** controls Metal

Table 6.1 The Five element correspondences: FIRE

The FIRE element		Huo xing 火行
FACULTY	Spiritual	: Shen, Spirit-Mind Consciousness
	Celestial Stems	: Bing (stem 3) and Ding (stem 4)
	Earthly branches	: Si (branch 6) and Wu (branch 7)
	Planet	: Mars
	Number	: 7
	Pentatonic note	: Zhi, (Lah, 5th or top note of scale)
	Genetic aspiration	: Realisation via love and self-reflection
	Cycle	: Growth
	Yin/Yang	: Utmost Yang
	Quality	: Radiating
ENVIRONMENTAL	Season	: Summer
	Phase of Moon	: Full moon decreasing to half moon
	Climate	: Hot
	Direction	: South
	Colour	: Red
	Part of the Day	: Noon
BODY	Organ Yin	: Heart
	Yang	: Small Intestine
	Tissue	: Blood Vessels
	Skin Colour	: Red, Purple
	Odour	: Burning
	Branch	: Facial Colour
	Sense Organ	: Tongue
	Senses	: Speech
	Fluid	: Sweat
EMOTIONAL	Emotion	: Joy, Hysteria
	Sound, Voice	: Laughing, Talkative
	Action	: Itching
FOOD (symbol)	Animal	: Sheep, Lamb
	Taste	: Bitter, Hot
	Fruit	: Apricot
	Grain	: Corn
	Vegetable	: Enlarged and Leafy (lettuce, cress, zucchini)

Heart Channel Points • Xin Jing Xue • 心經穴

IDENTIFICATION	ACTION	INDICATIONS
HT-1 Jiquan 極泉 Supreme Spring At the centre of the ARMPIT on the medial side of the AXILLARY ARTERY	Nourishes Heart Yin Clears Empty Fire Relaxes Chest and Shoulder	Dry mouth, night sweating, mental restlessness and insomnia Chest and cardiac pain Shoulder problems and arm pain
HT-3 Shaohai 少海 Lesser Yin Sea At the medial end of the transverse CUBITAL crease in the depression anterior to the MEDIAL EPICONDYLE of the HUMERUS *He-SEA POINT* *WATER POINT of the Heart channel*	Clears Heat Calms the Mind Removes obstructions from Channel	Insomnia Epilepsy Dizziness Depression Restlessness and forgetfulness Arm, chest and elbow pain
HT-7 Shenmen 神門 Spirit Gate On the transverse WRIST crease on the RADIAL side of the FLEXOR CARPI ULNARIS muscle. *Yuan-SOURCE POINT* *Shu-STREAM POINT* *EARTH POINT of the Heart channel*	Nourishes Heart Blood Calms the Mind	Asthmatic wheezing Hypertension Chest pain with palpitations Iinsomnia Poor memory Pale tongue Dizziness
HT-9 Shaochong 少衝 Lesser Rushing About 0.1 CUN from the RADIAL corner of the 5th FINGERNAIL, level with the base line of the nail. *Ying-WELL POINT* *WOOD POINT of the Heart channel*	Clears Heat Opens Heart orifices Restores consciousness	Anxiety Hysteria Hypomania, Chest pain due to emotional stress Coma Sudden loss of consciousness

Small Intestine Channel Points • Xiao Chang Jing Xue • 小腸經穴

IDENTIFICATION	ACTION	INDICATIONS
SI-1 Shaoze 少澤 Lesser Marsh About 0.1 CUN from the ULNAR corner of the 5th FINGERNAIL, level with the base line of the nail. *Jing-WELL POINT* *METAL POINT of the Small intestine channel*	Expels Wind-Heat (Exterior invasion) Opens Orifices Removes Channel obstructions Promotes Lactation	Stiff neck, headache, acute tonsillitis Deafness, tinnitus, and tongue stiffness Acute or chronic neck problems Mastitis and insufficient lactation
SI-3 Houxi 後谿 Back Stream At the medial end of the transverse CUBITAL crease in the depression anterior to the MEDIAL EPICONDYLE of the HUMERUS *Shu-STREAM POINT* *WOOD POINT of the Small intestine channel* *OPENING POINT of the Supervisor vessel*	Eliminates Interior Wind from Supervisor vessel Expels Exterior Wind Resolves Dampness Benefits Sinews Clears the Mind	Convulsions, tremors, epilepsy, stiff neck, dizziness and headache Stiff neck, occipital headache, spinal aches and fever and chills Jaundice and heaviness in the chest Acute upper back pain along the Small Intestine, Bladder channels and the Du mai (Supervisor vessel) Tendency for detailed thinking resulting in indecisiveness
SI-8 Xiaohai 小海 Small Sea With the ELBOW flexed, in the posterior aspect of the CUBITAL joint, in the FOSSA between the ULNAR OLECRANON and the MEDIAL EPICONDYLE of the HUMERUS *He-SEA POINT* *EARTH POINT of the Small intestine channel*	Resolves Damp Heat Removes Channel obstructions Calms the Mind	Acute swelling of the neck glands Elbow and neck pain Anxiety
SI-9 Jianzhen 肩貞 Upright Shoulder With the ARM at the side, located 1 CUN superior to the posterior end of the AXILLARY fold	Removes Channel obstructions	Pain, stiffness in shoulder, scapula or arm

Small Intestine Channel Points • Xiao Chang Jing Xue • 小腸經穴

IDENTIFICATION	ACTION	INDICATIONS
SI-10 Naoshu 臑俞 Upper Arm Shu With the ARM at the side, located directly superior to SI-9 Jianzhen in the depression inferior and lateral to the SCAPULAR SPINE.	Removes Channel obstructions	Frozen shoulder Pain, stiffness in shoulder, scapula or arm
SI-11 Tianzong 天宗 Heavenly Worship On the SCAPULA, in a depression located one third of the distance between the midpoint of the lower border of the SCAPULAR SPINE, and the inferior angle of the SCAPULA.	Removes Channel obstructions Relaxes Chest	Pain, stiffness in shoulder, scapula or arm Asthma Cough
SI-19 Tinggong 聽宮 Palace of Hearing With the MOUTH slightly opened, located in the depression between the TRAGUS and the MANDIBULAR joint. *MEETING POINT of the Small Intestine, Gall Bladder and Triple Heater channels*	Benefits the Ears Calms the Spirit	Deafness, tinnitus, all ear disorders Mania

Table 6.2 Functions of the Zang Fu (organ) and Zen Shiatsu (meridian) systems

ZANG FU 臟腑	HEART organ Xin zang 心臟	SMALL INTESTINE organ Xiao Chang fu 小腸腑
	Governs Blood (XUE) Controls the Blood Vessels (XUEMAI) Manifests in the Complexion Opens into the Tongue Controls Sweat Houses the Spirit-Mind (SHEN)	Seperates Pure from Impure Foods and Fluids for Absorption and Transformation
IMAGE	The **Monarch** who rules through insight and understanding	The **Official** in charge of screening substances for nourishment and transformation
GOVERNMENT	**KING**	**KINGS SECRETARY**

ZEN SHIATSU 神指士	HEART meridian Xin jing 心經	SMALL INTESTINE meridian Xiao Chang jing 小腸經
	Centre of Emotional response/reaction Governs Central Nervous Systems (CNS) Controls Blood Circulation and assists Immune System Represents Awareness and Compassion	Digests and assimilates Food from the Jejunem through the Ileum to the Ileocaecal Valve Produces Blood Maintains Composure through Shock Mechanism (Blood, CSF, Ovaries, Testes)
BASIC	Environmental Interpretation for Body Spirit-Mind	Conversion and Integration of Nurturing Substances
SPECIFIC	**EMOTIONAL CENTRE**	**ASSIMILATION**
GENERAL	**CONTROL**	

Table 6.3 Zen Shiatsu correspondences: Heart meridian

HEART meridian			Xin jing 心經
FACULTY	Spiritual Input	:	SHEN, Spirit-Mind
	Functions via	:	Conciousness
	Represents	:	Awareness
	Supplemented by	:	Emotional Centre
	Realised by	:	Guiding
	Dominant Zone	:	Inside
	Embryological Layer	:	Endoderm
	Meridian Nature	:	Yin
	Tuning Time	:	11am - 1pm
ANATOMY & PHYSIOLOGY	Brain	]	Central Nervous system
	Spinal Cord	]	Senso-Physical Initiative
	Eyes	]	Speech
	Tongue	]	
	Thymus Gland	]	Immune system
		]	'T' Cells Lymphocytes
	Heart	]	Circulatory System
	Sino-atrial Node	]	Blood Circulation
	Atrio-ventricular node	]	
PHYSICAL	Angina Pectoris		Myocardial Infarction
	Asthma		Oedema
	Blood Pressure Problems		Palmar Sweats
	Cardiac Arrhythmias		Palpitations
	Chest Stiffness		Poor Circulation
	Corner of Eyes - Red		Red Complexion
	Endocarditis		Rheumatic Fever
	Epigastric Tightness		Speech Problems
	Excessive Sweating		Swallowing Difficulties
	Fatigue after Exertion		Tongue Stiffness
PSYCHOLOGICAL	Adaptory Issues		Manipulative
	Anxiety		Memory Problems
	Emotional Tiredness		Nervousness
	Emotional Trauma		Neurotic
	Erratic Behaviour		Perpetual Fatigue
	Excessive Laughter		Restlessness
	Hand Tension		Stammering
	Hysteria		Talkative
	Lack of Compassion		Thirst
	Low Spirit		Worry

Table 6.4 Zen Shiatsu correspondences: Small Intestine meridian

SMALL INTESTINE meridian		Xiao Chang jing 小腸經
FACULTY	Spiritual Input	: SHEN via Heart meridian
	Functions via	: Conciousness
	Represents	: Absorption
	Supplemented by	: Assimilation
	Realised by	: Experiencing
	Dominant Zone	: Inside
	Embryological Layer	: Endoderm
	Meridian Nature	: Yang
	Tuning Time	: 1pm - 3pm
ANATOMY & PHYSIOLOGY	Brain]	Cerebrospinal Fluid (CSF)
	Spinal Cord]	
	Small Intestine (Ileum)]	Digestive System
	]	Blood Quality
	Ovaries]	Hormonal System
	Testes]	Reproductive System
PHYSICAL	Anaemia	Hearing Disorders
	Appendicitis	Hip Pain, Sciatica
	Blood Disorders	Lordosis & Lumbar Pain
	Borborygmi	Malabsorption
	Chilly Extremities	Menstrual Problems
	Constipation	Migraine Headaches
	Diarrhoea	Neck & Back Stiffness
	Ear & Jaw Pain	Physical Injury, Trauma
	Enteritis & Fever	Reproductive Problems
	Fatigued Easily	Toothache
PSYCHOLOGICAL	Acceptance	Overdetermination
	Concentration	Over Focused
	Confidence Issues	Patience
	Discriminate Nature	Restless
	Emotional Trauma	Righteous
	Experimentation	Selfish
	Indecisive	Shock
	Judgemental	Sorrowful
	Lack of Reality	Suppression of Feelings
	Obsession with Small Details	Wanting It All

Fig. 6.2 Anterior upper view: Zen Shiatsu Heart and Small Intestine meridians

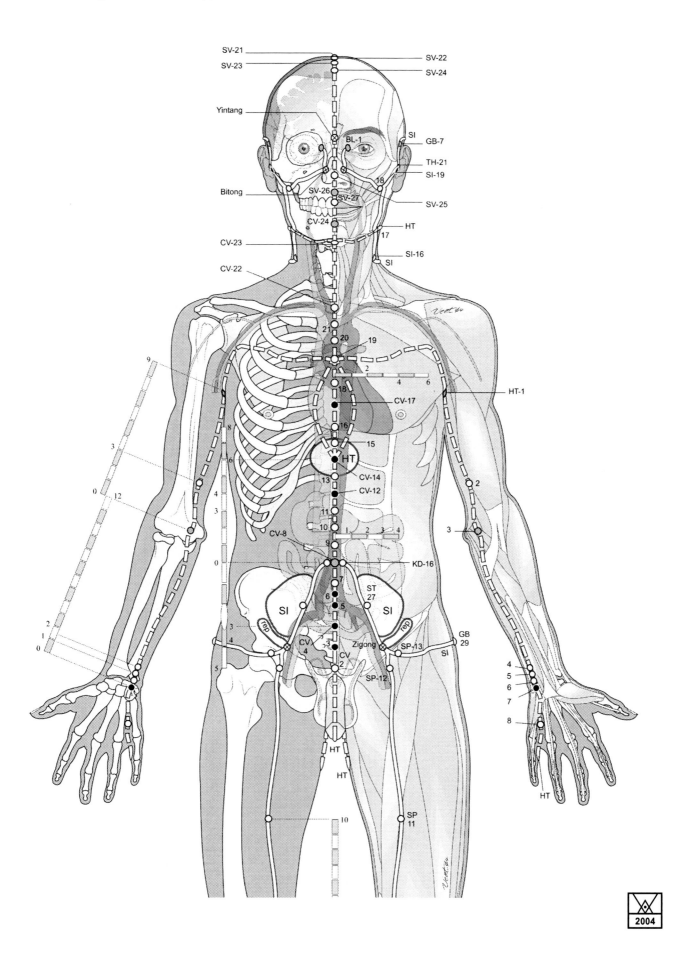

Fig. 6.3 Anterior lower view: Zen Shiatsu Heart and Small Intestine meridians

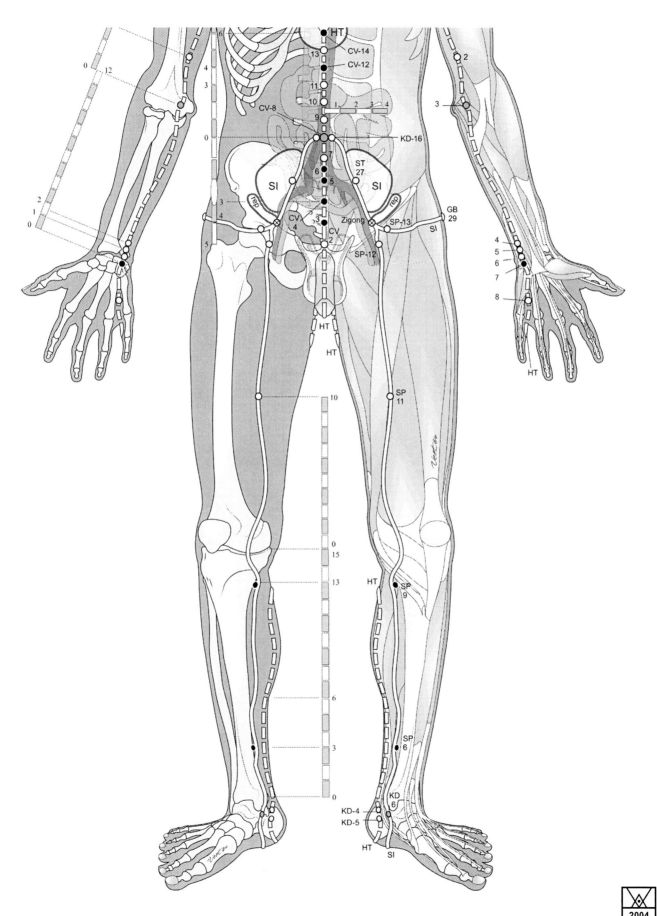

Fig. 6.4 Posterior upper view: Zen Shiatsu Heart and Small Intestine meridians

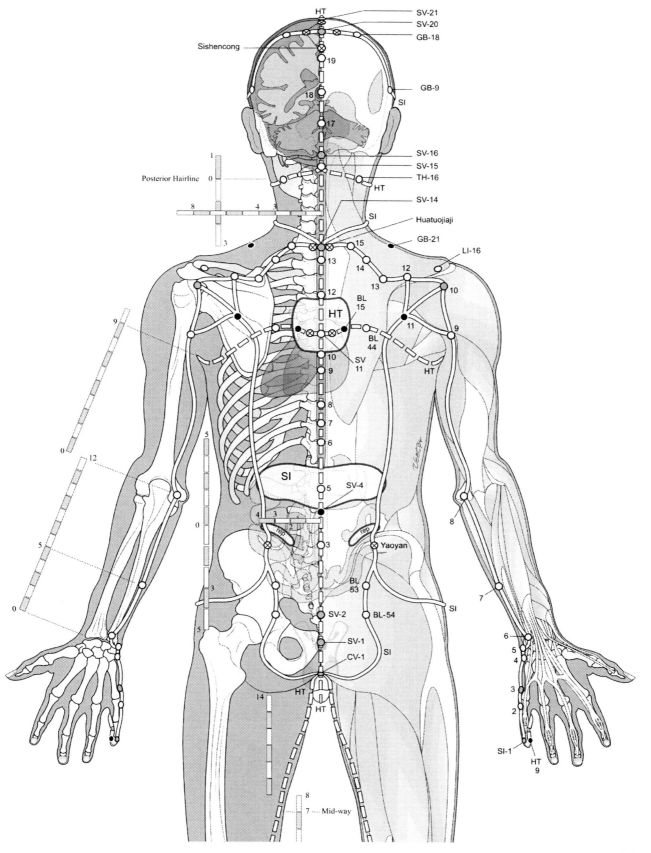

Fig. 6.5 Posterior lower view: Zen Shiatsu Heart and Small Intestine meridians

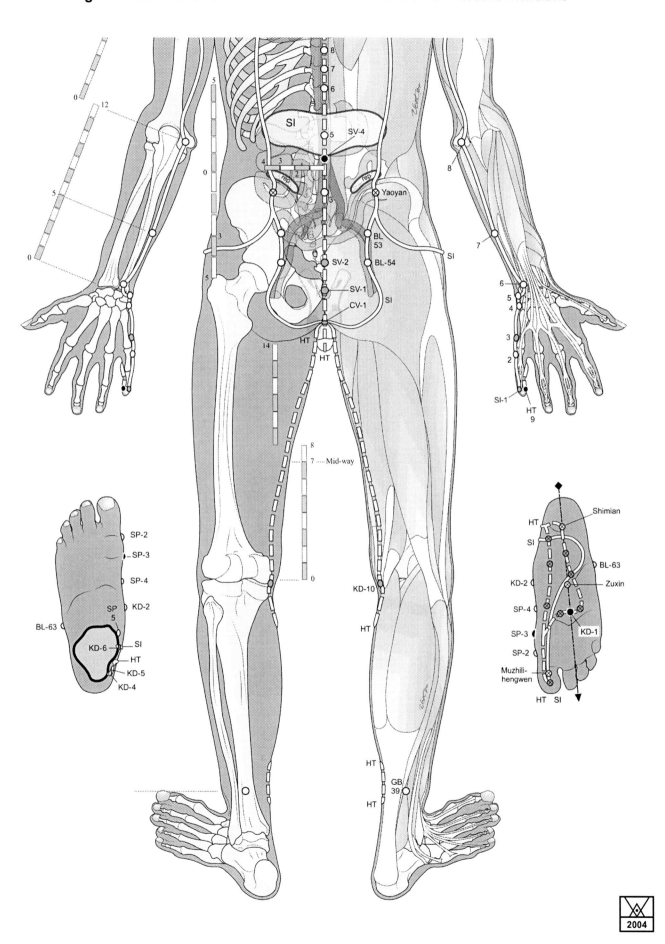

Fig. 6.6 Head cranial and lateral details: Zen Shiatsu Heart and Small Intestine meridians

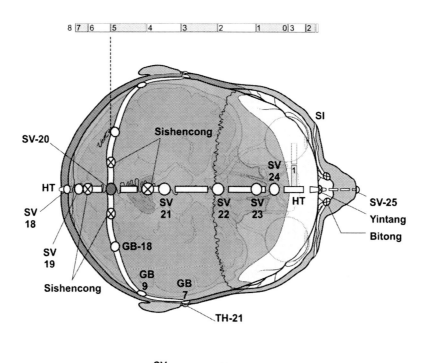

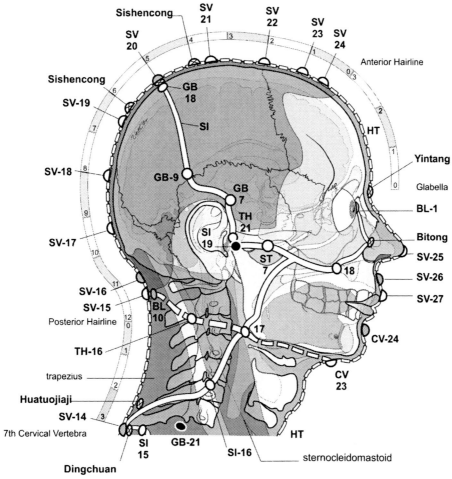

Fig. 6.7 Lower Arm and Hand details: Zen Shiatsu Heart and Small Intestine meridians

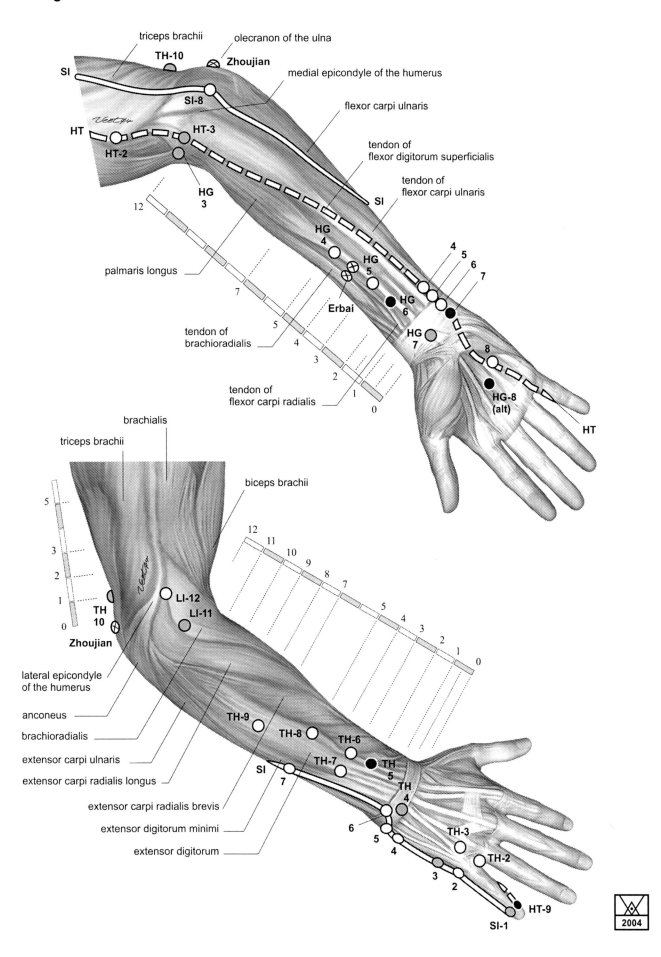

Fig. 6.8 Male Perineum details: Zen Shiatsu Heart and Small Intestine meridians

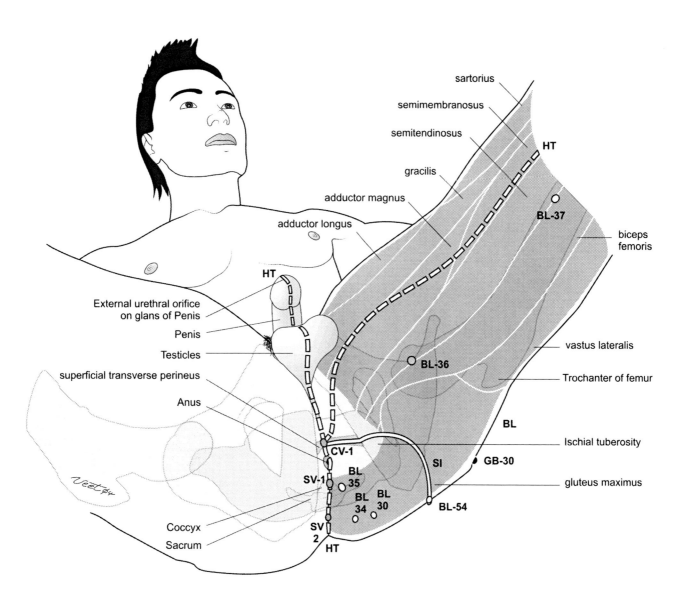

Fig. 6.9 Female Perineum details: Zen Shiatsu Heart and Small Intestine meridians

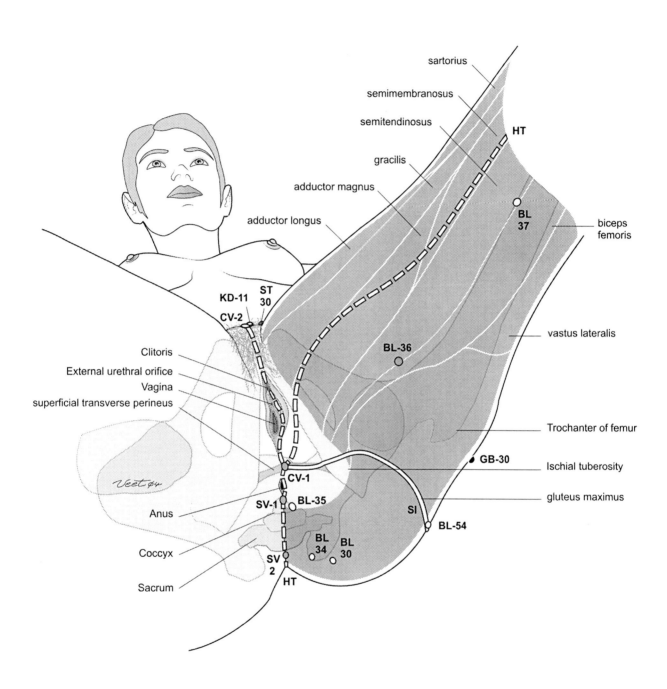

Fig. 6.10 Lower Leg and Foot details: Zen Shiatsu Heart and Small Intestine meridians

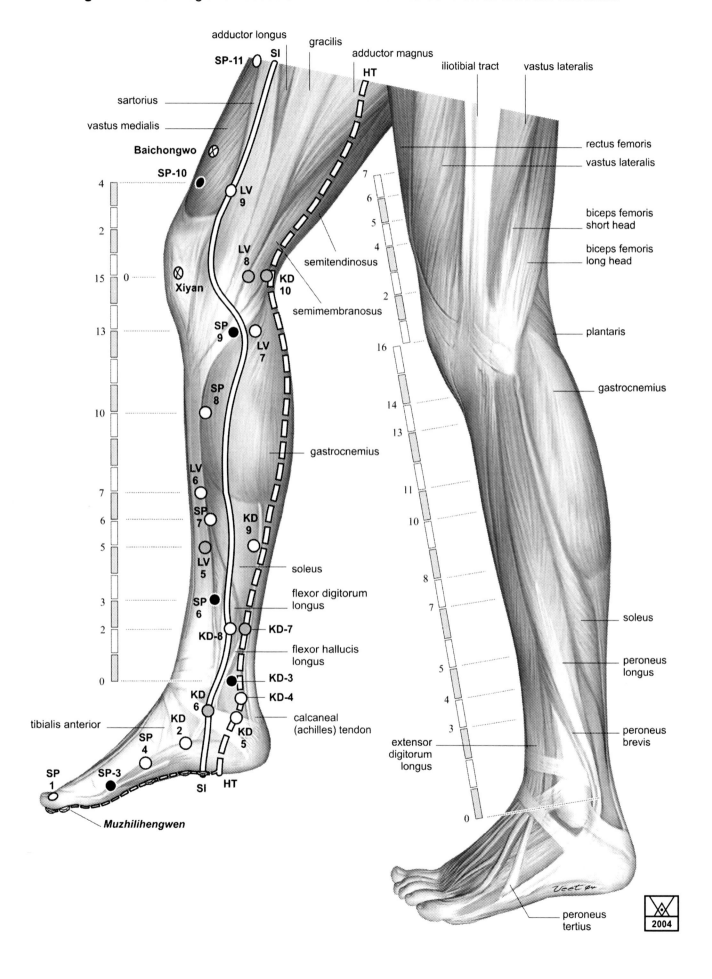

Fig. 6.11 Foot dorsal and plantar details: Zen Shiatsu Heart and Small Intestine meridians

Foot: Dorsal view

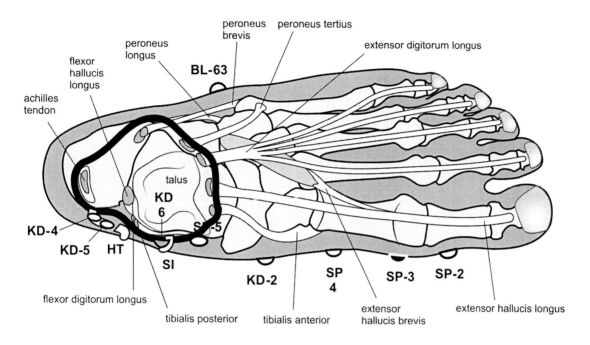

Foot: Plantar view

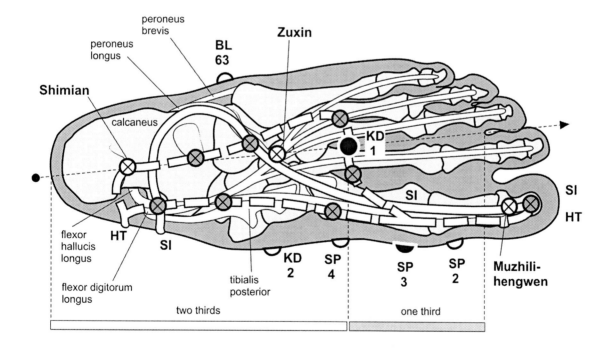

Chapter 7
the FIRE element part two

Heart Governor
and
Triple Heater

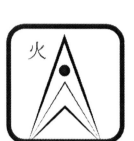

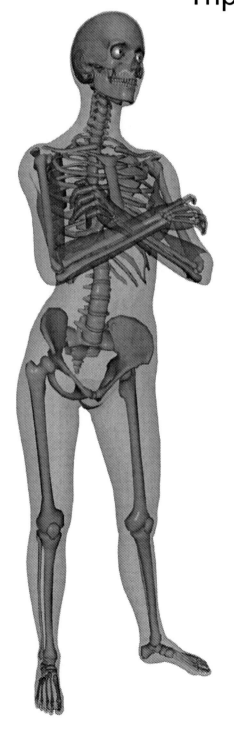

Fig. 7.1 The Five element sequences: FIRE

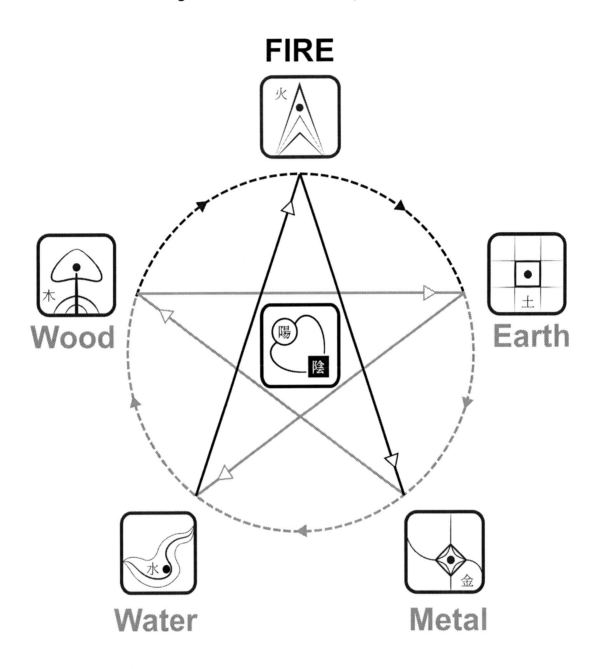

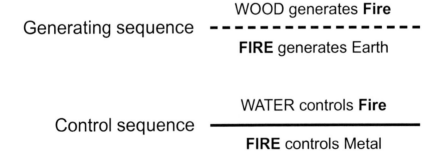

Table 7.1 The Five element correspondences: FIRE

The FIRE element		Huo xing 火行
FACULTY	Spiritual	: Shen, Spirit-Mind Consciousness
	Celestial Stems	: Bing (stem 3) and Ding (stem 4)
	Earthly branches	: Si (branch 6) and Wu (branch 7)
	Planet	: Mars
	Number	: 7
	Pentatonic note	: Zhi, (Lah, 5th or top note of scale)
	Genetic aspiration	: Realisation via love and self-reflection
	Cycle	: Growth
	Yin/Yang	: Utmost Yang
	Quality	: Radiating
ENVIRONMENTAL	Season	: Summer
	Phase of Moon	: Full moon decreasing to half moon
	Climate	: Hot
	Direction	: South
	Colour	: Red
	Part of the Day	: Noon
BODY	Organ Yin	: supplementary (Heart Governor)
	Yang	: supplementary (Triple Heater)
	Tissue	: Blood Vessels
	Skin Colour	: Red, Purple
	Odour	: Burning
	Branch	: Facial Colour
	Sense Organ	: Tongue
	Senses	: Speech
	Fluid	: Sweat
EMOTIONAL	Emotion	: Joy, Hysteria
	Sound, Voice	: Laughing, Talkative
	Action	: Itching
FOOD (symbol)	Animal	: Sheep, Lamb
	Taste	: Bitter, Hot
	Fruit	: Apricot
	Grain	: Corn
	Vegetable	: Enlarged and Leafy (lettuce, cress, zucchini)

Heart Governor Channel Points • Xin Zhu Jing Xue • 心主經穴

IDENTIFICATION	ACTION	INDICATIONS
HG-1 Tianchi 天池 Heavenly Pool 1 CUN lateral to the NIPPLE, in the 4th INTERCOSTAL SPACE. *MEETING POINT of the Heart Governor, Triple Heater, Gall Bladder and the Liver channels*	Clears stagnant Liver Qi	Chest fullness Hypochondriac pain (under ribs)
HG-3 Quze 曲澤 Crooked marsh With the ELBOW flexed, on the transverse CUBITAL crease, on the ULNAR side of the TENDON of the BICEPS BRACHII muscle. *He-SEA POINT* *WATER POINT of the Heart Governor channel*	Clears Heat Cools Blood Calms the Mind	Heatstroke Inflammation of Stomach or Intestines Skin eruptions Fever Severe anxiety Palpitations
HG-6 Neiguan 內関 Inner Pass 2 CUN proximal to HM-7 Daling (at the transverse WRIST crease) between the TENDONS of the PALMARIS LONGUS and FLEXOR CARPI RADIALIS muscles. *Luo-CONNECTING POINT* *OPENING POINT of the Yin Tie vessel*	Opens the Chest Subdues rebellious Stomach Qi Calms the Mind	All chest problems Stagnant type chest pain Nausea and vomiting Travel sickness Stomach pain Heartburn, hiccup and belching Irritability and anxiety Pre-menstrual pain Depression and restlessness
HG-7 Daling 大陵 Great Mound At the transverse crease of the WRIST, between the TENDONS of the PALMARIS LONGUS and FLEXOR CARPI RADIALIS muscles, level with the proximal border of the PISIFORM bone. *Yuan-SOURCE POINT* *Shu-STREAM POINT* *EARTH POINT of the Heart Governor channel* *Sun Si-miao GHOST POINT*	Calms the Mind Clears Heat and cools the Blood Harmonises the Stomach Relaxes the Chest	Emotional difficulties Anxiety, excessive laughter and mania, mental reslessness, fright, sadness, panic Fever with or without sweating Dry throat, pain at the root of the tongue Acute headache, red eyes Skin rashes, acne, hand eczema Acute vomiting Stomach pain Pain or swelling of the Chest including the side and armpit areas Breathlessness

Heart Governor Channel Points • Xin Zhu Jing Xue • 心主經穴

IDENTIFICATION	ACTION	INDICATIONS
HG-8 Laogong 籂宮 Palace of Toil On the palm, on the RADIAL side of the 3rd METACARPAL bone, proximal to the METACARPO PHALANGEAL joint. *Ying-SPRING POINT* *FIRE POINT of the Heart Governor channel* *Sun Si-miao GHOST POINT*	Clears Heart Fire Calms the Mind	Mental symptoms High fever and delirium Excessive thirst Tongue ulcers Restlessness Emotional pain
HG-9 Zhongchong 中衝 Central Thoroughfare At the centre of the tip of the middle FINGER. *Jing-WELL POINT* *WOOD POINT of the Heart Governor channel*	Clears Heat Expels Wind Restores consciousness	Mental symptoms Heatstroke Chest or gastric pain Loss of consciousness

心主經穴

Triple Heater Channel Points • San Jiao Jing Xue • 三焦經穴

IDENTIFICATION	ACTION	INDICATIONS
TH-1 Guanchong 關衝 Rushing Pass About 0.1 CUN from the lateral corner of the 4th FINGERNAIL, level with the base line of the nail. *Jing-WELL POINT* *METAL POINT of the Triple Heater channel*	Clears Heat Expels Wind Restores consciousness Removes Channel obstructions	Fever Sore throat Earache Loss of consciousness Painful and stiff shoulder joint
TH-4 Yangchi 陽池 Yang Pool In a depression of the transverse dorsal crease of the WRIST between the TENDONS of the EXTENSOR DIGITORUM and EXTENSOR DIGITI MINIMI muscles. *Yuan-SOURCE POINT*	Relaxes Sinews Clears Heat	Occipital headache Neck, shoulder, arm or wrist pain Painful obstruction of the throat Dry mouth and thirst Fever without sweat Malaria
TH-5 Waiguan 外関 Outer Pass 2 CUN above the dorsal WRIST crease between the RADIUS and the ULNA, on the radial side of the EXTENSOR DIGITORUM muscle. *Luo-CONNECTING POINT* *OPENING POINT of the Yang Tie vessel*	Expels External Wind-Heat Removes Channel obstructions Benefits the Ear Subdues Liver Yang	Fever, sore throat, slight sweating Aversion to cold Pain in the arm, shoulder, neck and hand Ear infection from Exterior Wind Heat Tinnitus or deafness from Liver Fire or Yang rising Migraine headaches on temples
TH-10 Tianjing 天井 Heavenly Well 1 CUN superior to the OLECRANON in the depression made by flexing the ELBOW *He-SEA POINT* *EARTH POINT of the Triple Heater channel*	Expels Wind Benefits the Eyes Stops Pain	Headache at outer corner of eyebrow (with Liver pattern) Any eye problems Headache on temples, facial paralysis at outer corner of eyebrow

Triple Heater Channel Points • San Jiao Jing Xue • 三焦經穴

IDENTIFICATION	ACTION	INDICATIONS
TH-14 Jianliao 肩髎 Shoulder Bone Hole With the arm abducted, located at the SHOULDER, in a depression formed between the posterior and inferior end of the ACROMION, and the GREATER TUBERCLE of the HUMERUS.	Removes Channel obstructions Resolves Dampness	Channel pain Painful elbow with stiff tendons Swelling of glands and tonsils from External Damp Heat
TH-23 Sizhukong 絲竹空 Silk Bamboo Hole On the lateral border of the SUPRA-ORBITAL margin, in a depression at the lateral tip of the EYEBROW	Expels Wind Benefits the Eyes Stops pain	Headache at outer corner of eyebrow (with Liver pattern) Any eye problems Headache on temples Facial paralysis at outer corner of eyebrow

Table 7.2 Functions of the Zang Fu (organ) and Zen Shiatsu (meridian) systems

ZANG FU 臟 腑	HEART GOVERNOR organ Xin Bao zang 心主臟	TRIPLE HEATER organ San Jiao fu 三焦腑
	Protects the Heart (XIN) Governs Blood (XUE) Controls the Blood Vessels (XUEMAI) Guides Joy and Pleasure	Regulates JINYE Metabolism
IMAGE	The **Palace Official** from whom pleasure and mirth are derived	The **Official** in charge of the Waterworks
GOVERNMENT	**KINGS AMBASSADOR**	**WATER ENGINEER**

ZEN SHIATSU 神 指 土	HEART GOVERNOR meridian Xin Zhu jing 心主經	TRIPLE HEATER meridian San Jiao jing 三焦經
	Governs the Vascular System and central Lymphatic Ducts Assists Heart control central Circulation Protects and assists Heart in Emotional response/reaction	Governs the Lymphatic System, Portal and Peripheral Circulation and Immune System Regulates the Distribution of Nutrients from the Mesentery to the Extremities Produces and regulates Heat via Metabolism Regulates Connective Tissue and Fascia
BASIC	Circulates Nutrients and vital Information for Life Process	Directs Nutrients and Instructions for Defence
SPECIFIC	**STABILISES BODY VIA VASCULAR RESPONSE**	**MAINTAINS BODY VIA LYMPHATIC RESPONSE**
GENERAL	**PROTECTION**	

Table 7.3 Zen Shiatsu correspondences: Heart Governor meridian

HEART GOVERNOR meridian		Xin Zhu jing 心主經
FACULTY	Spiritual Input	: SHEN, via Heart Meridian
	Functions via	: Conciousness
	Represents	: Interpretation
	Supplemented by	: Vascular Response
	Realised by	: Communicating
	Dominant Zone	: Surface
	Embryological Layer	: Ectoderm
	Meridian Nature	: Yin
	Tuning Time	: 7pm - 9pm
ANATOMY & PHYSIOLOGY	Meninges	] Central Nervous system (CNS)
	Pericardium	] Systemic & Pulmonary
	Heart	] Circulation
	Aorta	]
	Major Arteries and Veins	]
	Thoracic & Right Lymphatic Ducts	] Lymphatic System
	Thymus	]
	Angina Pectoris	Palpitations
	Blood Pressure Disorders	Pins & Needles
	Chest Pain, Stiffness	Poor Working Posture
	Circulatory Disorders	Pulse Irregulaties
	Cold Extremeties	Pyloric Pain, Stiffness
	Head Haziness	Pyrosis (Heartburn)
	Heart Disorders	Throat Inflammation/Fever
	Insomnia	Tiredness on Exertion
	Meningitis	Tonsilitis
	Oedema	Wheezing
PSYCHOLOGICAL	Absent Minded	Lack of Reality
	Breathing Difficulties	Negotiative
	Can't Explain Things	Obsessed with Moving Things
	Disturbed Sleep	Oppressive Feeling in Chest
	Easily Startled	Overactive
	Emotional Trauma	Overfocused on Work
	Excessive Dreaming	Relationship Issues
	Hypersensitive	Restlessness
	Inability to Relax	Social Nervousness
	Joyfullness	Stability Issues

Table 7.4 Zen Shiatsu correspondences: Triple Heater meridian

TRIPLE HEATER meridian		San Jiao jing 三焦經
FACULTY	Spiritual Input	: SHEN via Heart meridian
	Functions via	: Conciousness
	Represents	: Maintenance
	Supplemented by	: Lymphatic Response
	Realised by	: Guarding
	Dominant Zone	: Surface
	Embryological Layer	: Ectoderm
	Meridian Nature	: Yang
	Tuning Time	: 9pm-11pm
ANATOMY & PHYSIOLOGY	Meninges	] Central Nervous System (CNS)
	Lymph Nodes, Tissues and	] Lymphatic System
	Vessels	] Immune response
	Spleen and Thymus	] Lymphocytes, Phago-cytosis
	Mucous, Serous Membranes	]
	Thyroid	] Thyroid Regulatory Metabolism
	Skin	] Connective tissue
	Fascia	] Peripheral Circulation
	Capillaries	]
	Cystic, Gastric, Mesentric, and Splenic Veins	] Portal Circulation
PHYSICAL	Allergies	Neck Pain
	Colds, Sneezing	Oedema
	Dizziness	Poor Circulation-Extremities
	Eczema, Urticaria	Psoriasis
	Excess Mucous Secretion	Sensitive Skin
	Eye, Throat Infections	Temperature Sensitivity
	Headaches	Sneezing
	Immune Deficiency	Swollen Lymph Glands/Nodes
	Meningitis	Tight Chest and Abdomen
	Nasal Problems	Tonsillitis
PSYCHOLOGICAL	Armouring (Body Mind)	Over Mothered
	Awkward Stance	Overly Cautious
	Burdened	Pretentious
	Confidence Issues	Protective Attitude
	Disorganised	Relationship problems
	Focused on Tiredness	Sensitive to Change
	Hardness	Social Problems
	Hides behind Others	Stunned
	Hypersensitive	Trauma
	Overactive	Unadventurous

Fig. 7.2 Anterior upper view: Zen Shiatsu Heart Governor and Triple Heater meridians

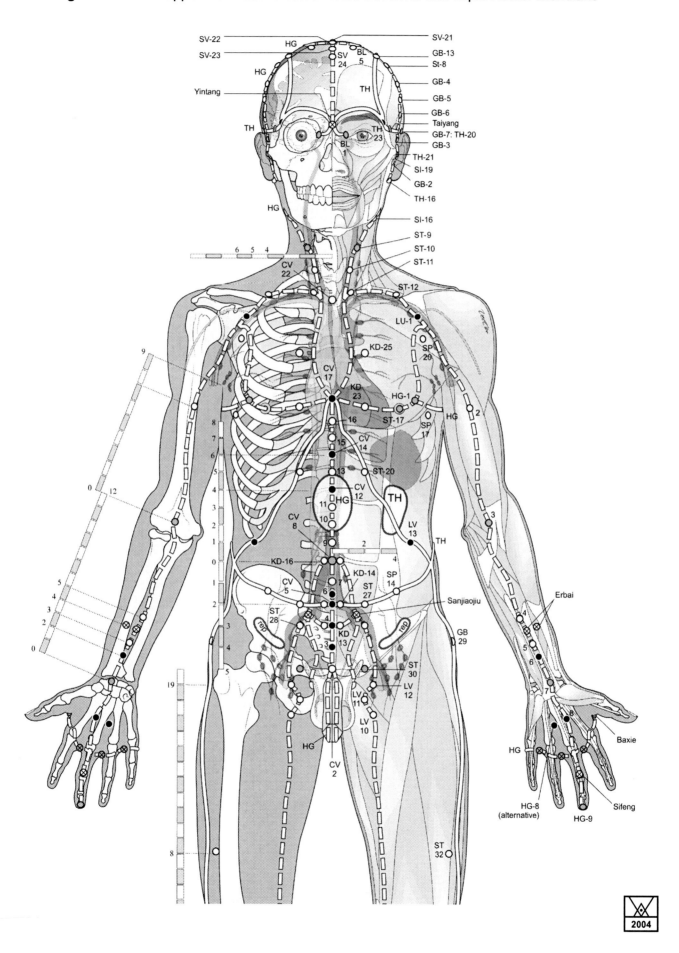

Fig. 7.3 Anterior lower view: Zen Shiatsu Heart Governor and Triple Heater meridians

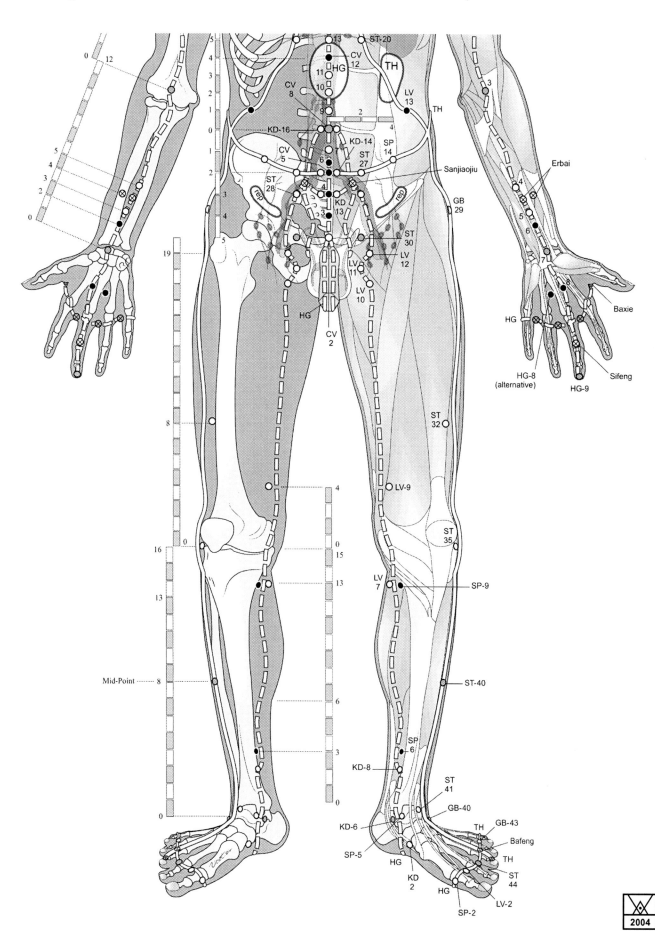

Fig. 7.4 Posterior upper view: Zen Shiatsu Heart Governor and Triple Heater meridians

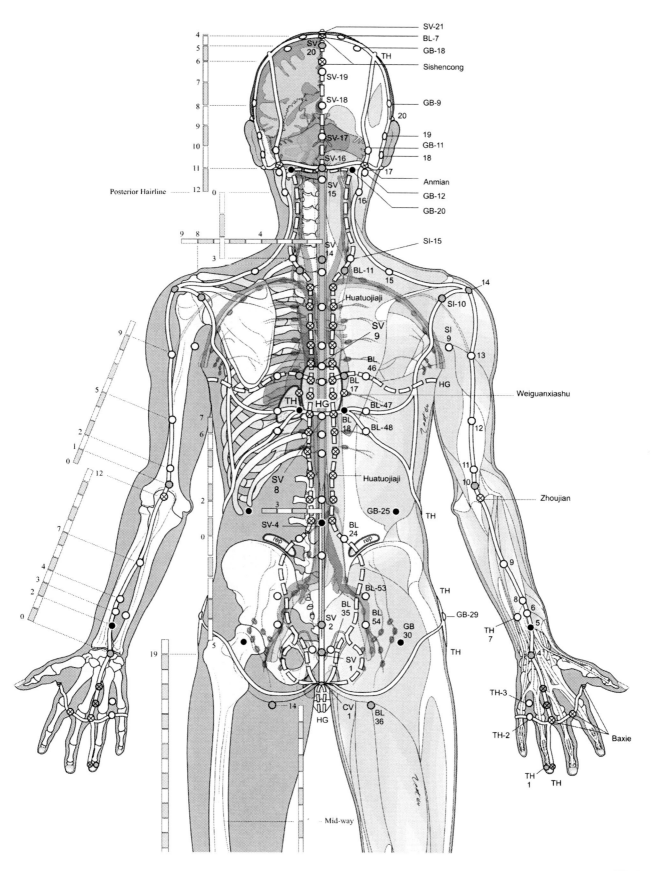

Fig. 7.5 Posterior lower view: Zen Shiatsu Heart Governor and Triple Heater meridians

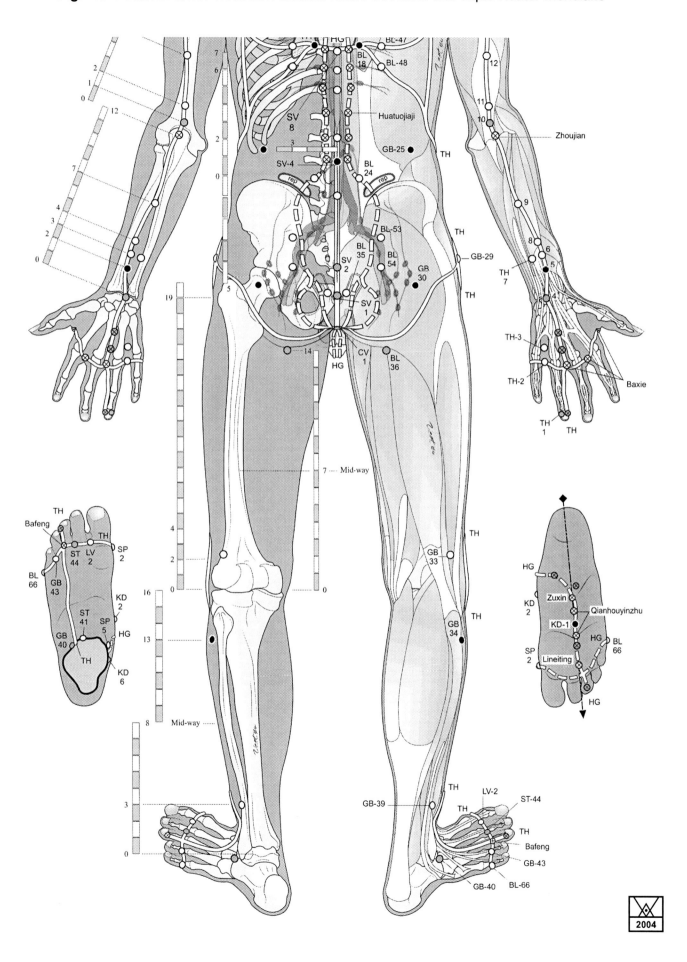

Fig. 7.6 Head cranial and lateral details: Zen Shiatsu Heart Governor and Triple Heater meridians

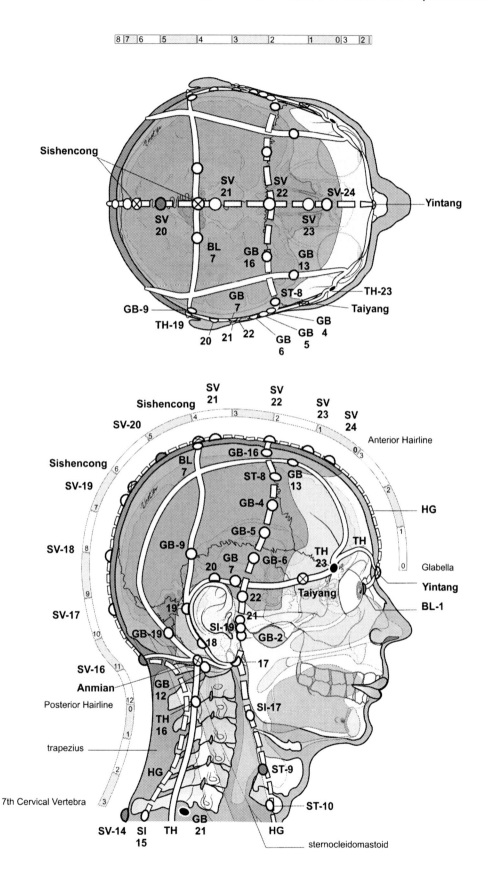

Fig. 7.7 Lower Arm and hand details: Zen Shiatsu Heart Governor and Triple Heater meridians

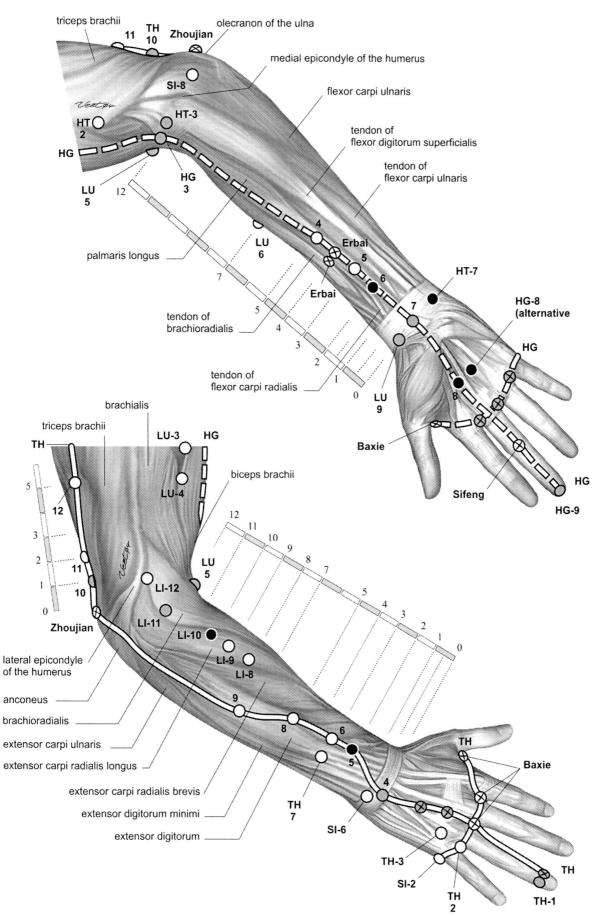

Fig. 7.8 Male Perineum details: Zen Shiatsu Heart Governor and Triple Heater meridians

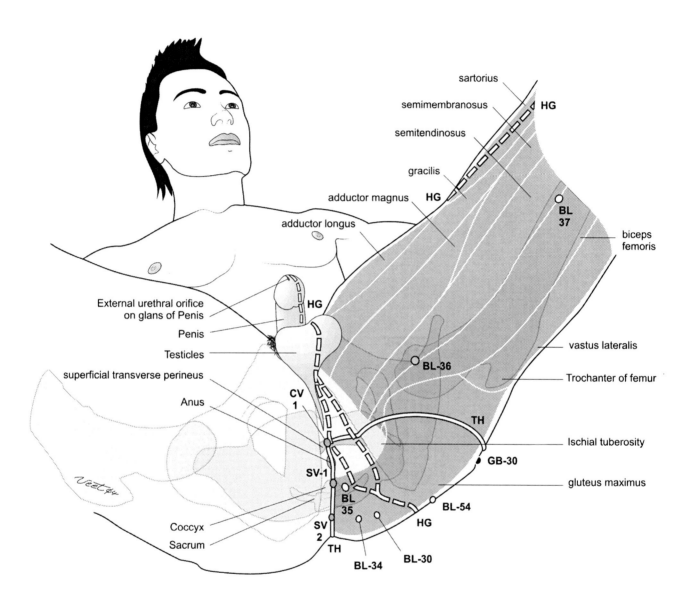

Fig. 7.9 Female Perineum details: Zen Shiatsu Heart Governor and Triple Heater meridians

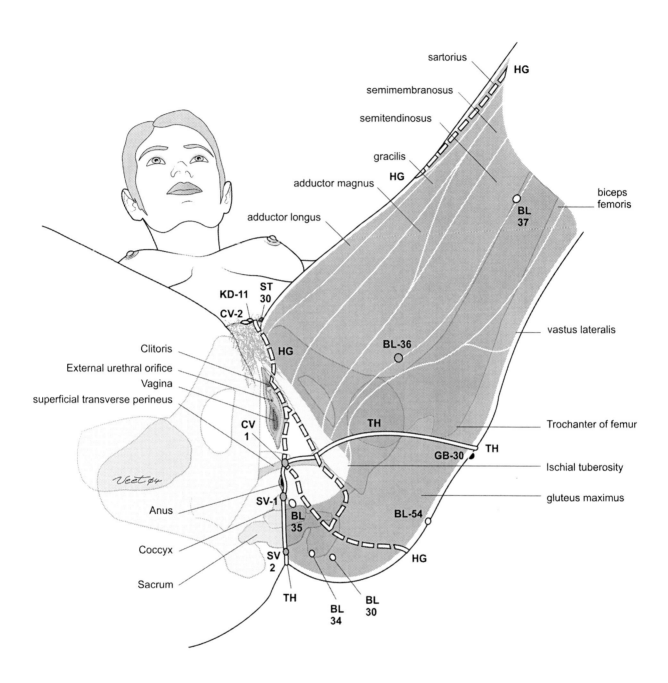

Fig. 7.10 Lower Leg and Foot details: Zen Shiatsu Heart Governor and Triple Heater meridians

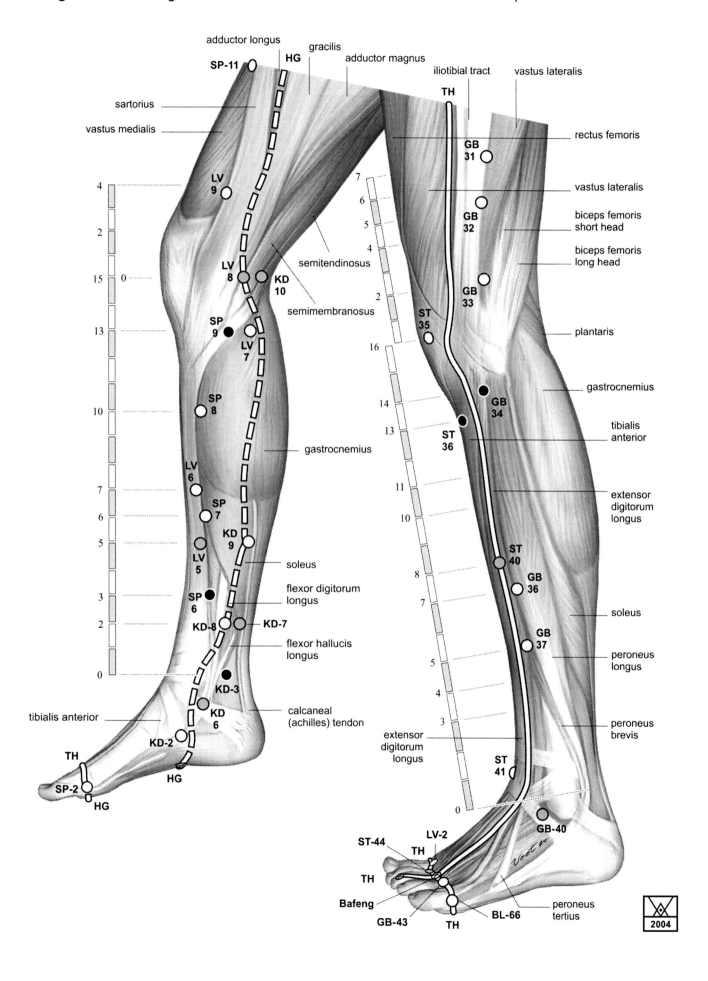

Fig. 7.11 Foot dorsal and plantar details: Zen Shiatsu Heart Governor and Triple Heater meridians

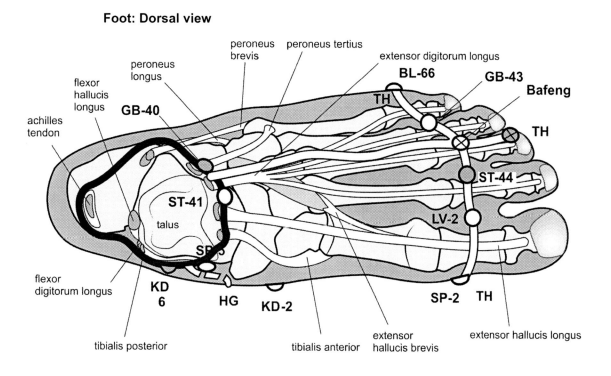

Foot: Dorsal view

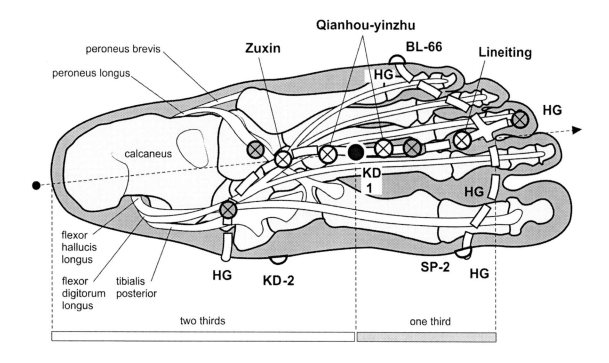

Foot: Plantar view

Chapter 8
the Earth element

Stomach
and
Spleen

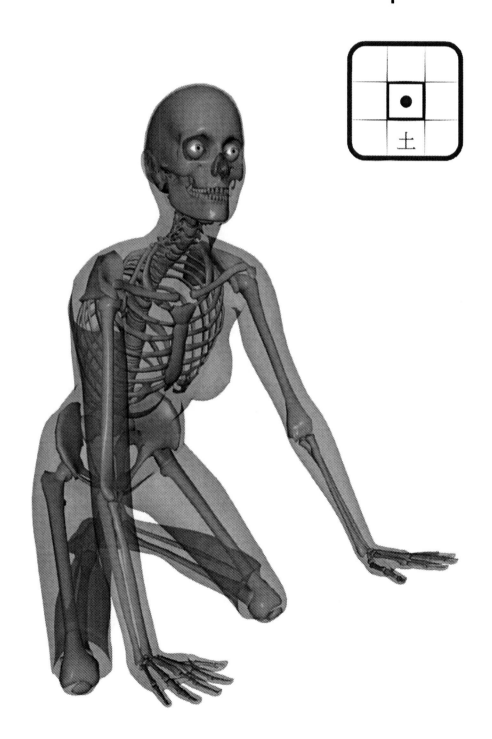

Fig. 8.1 The Five element sequences: EARTH

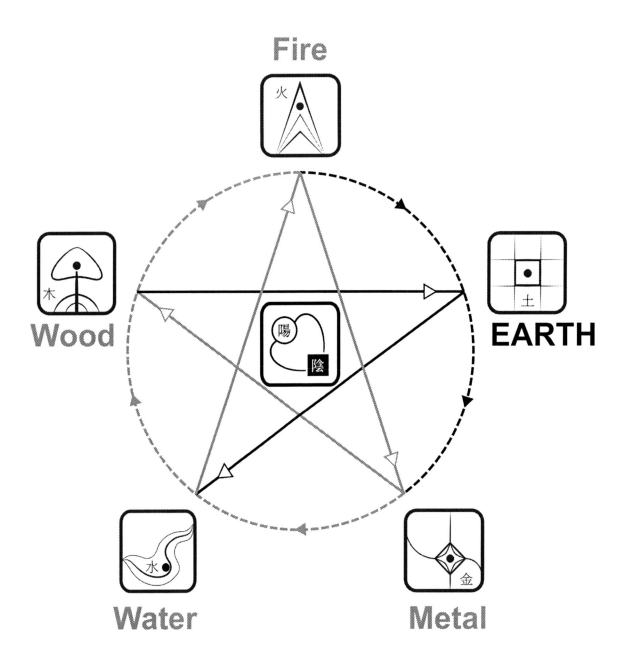

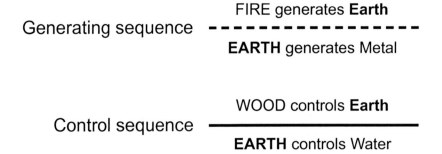

Generating sequence

FIRE generates **Earth**

EARTH generates Metal

Control sequence

WOOD controls **Earth**

EARTH controls Water

Table 8.1 The Five element correspondences: EARTH

The EARTH element		Tu xing 土行
FACULTY	Spiritual	: Y i, Thought Intellect
	Celestial Stem	: Wu (stem 5) and Ji (stem 6)
	Earthly branches	: Chou (branch 2), Chen (branch 5), Wei (branch 8) and Xu (branch 9)
	Planet	: Saturn
	Number	: 5
	Pentatonic note	: Gong, (Doh, base note of scale)
	Genetic aspiration	: Materialisation via nourishment
	Cycle	: Maturity
	Yin/Yang	: Centre
	Quality	: Downward, Stillness
ENVIRONMENTAL	Season	: Late Summer, Links each season to next
	Phase of Moon	: None, Links each phase to next
	Climate	: Damp, Humid
	Direction	: Centre
	Colour	: Yellow
	Part of the Day	: Afternoon
BODY	Organ Yin	: Spleen (Pancreas)
	Yang	Stomach
	Tissue	: Muscle, Flesh
	Skin Colour	: Yellow, Brown
	Odour	: Fragrant
	Branch	: Lips
	Sense Organ	: Mouth
	Senses	: Taste
	Fluid	: Sticky Saliva
EMOTIONAL	Emotion	: Empathy, Meditative thought
	Sound, Voice	: Singing, Lilting
	Action	: Belching
FOOD (symbol)	Animal	: Ox/Cow (Beef)
	Taste	: Sweet
	Fruit	: Dates
	Grain	: Millet
	Vegetable	: Round and Sweet (carrots, parsnips, turnip)

Stomach Channel Points • Wei Jing Xue • 胃經穴

IDENTIFICATION	ACTION	INDICATIONS
ST-1 Chengqi 承泣 Container of Tears Located directly inferior to the PUPIL on the inferior ridge of the ORBITAL CAVITY **** Moxibustion is contra-indicated ****	Expels Wind (Int and Ext) Brightens the Eyes	Facial swelling, pain, conjunctivitis and paralysis of eyelid Redness, colour and night blindness Wasting of optic nerve
ST-3 巨髎 Juliao Big Bone Located directly inferior to ST-1 Chengqi at the level of the inferior border of the ALA NASI	Expels Wind (Int and Ext) Relieves swelling Removes Channel obstructions	As ST--1 Chengqi above Also facial paralysis and trigeminal neuralgia Nasal obstruction, toothache and lip pain
ST-9 Renying 人迎 Human's Welcome At the level of the LARYNGEAL prominence, located on the anterior border of the STERNO-CLEIDO-MASTOID muscle where the pulse of the COMMON CAROTID ARTERY can be felt. *SEA of QI POINT* *MEETING POINT of the Stomach and Gall Bladder channels* *WINDOW of HEAVEN POINT* **** Moxibustion is contra-indicated **** **** Proceed with caution if blood pressure extremely high especially in early stages of cerebro vascular accident (CVA) ****	Regulates Qi and Blood Diffuses Lung Qi Benefits and moistens the Throat Stops pain Softens hard masses, resolves swellings	High or low blood pressure Hypertension Asthma, wheezing, belching, hiccup and nausea Oesophageal constriction with inability to swallow Sore throat, swollen larynx Acute obstruction of channels due to trauma (particularly lower back) Goitre (thyroid enlargement), pharyngitis (inflammation of rear cavity of the mouth) and tonsillitis

Stomach Channel Points • Wei Jing Xue • 胃經穴

IDENTIFICATION	ACTION	INDICATIONS
ST-17 Ruzhong 乳中 Breast Centre Located in the centre of the NIPPLE in the 4th INTERCOSTAL SPACE (between the 4th and 5th RIBS), 4 SUN lateral to the Controller Vessel. **** Acupuncture and Moxibustion contra-indicated **** **** Breast Area contra-indicated if cancer or inflammation are present ****	Mainly used as a reference point to locate points in the Chest and Abdomen Insufficient Lactation ** Local point ST-18 Rugen (Breast Centre) is preferred for Breast problems, especially in women **	A method of promoting lactation by massage is outlined in page 212 of the book "Tsubo" by Serizawa, Katsusuke., Japan Publications inc, Tokyo, New York, 1976.
ST-25 Tianshu 天樞 Heaven's Pivot 2 CUN lateral to the centre of the UMBILICUS, level with CV-8 Shenque. *FRONT Mu-COLLECTING POINT of the Large Intestine channel*	Regulates Intestinal functioning Relieves food retention Clears Heat (Intestines and Stomach)	Abdominal swelling, constipation, intestine pain Epigastric burning sensation, constipation, thirst, foul smelling loose stools or chronic diarrhoea, mental irritation
ST-30 Qichong 氣衝 Qi Thoroughfare 2 CUN lateral to the midline or the Controller vessel, level with CV-2 Qugu and the superior ridge of the PUBIC SYMPHYSIS. *SEA of FOOD POINT* *MEETING POINT of the Stomach channel and the Through-way vessel* *POINT of the Through-way vessel*	Regulates Qi Regulates Blood Regulates the Chong mai (Through-way vessel) Promotes Essence	Abdominal pain, heat or cold. Hernia Pain and swelling of the external genitals (vagina, penis or testicles) Retention of placenta. Retention of urine Foetal Qi ascending to harass the Heart (of the mother) Irregular, painful menstruation due to blood stasis. Absence of menses Uterine bleeding and childbirth disorders Infertility, impotence
ST-34 Liangqiu 梁丘 Beam Mound Located 2 CUN superior to the lateral superior border of the PATELLA *Xi-ACCUMULATING POINT*	Regulates Stomach Qi Removes Channel obstructions Expels Dampness and Wind	Acid regurgitation, stomach ache and nausea, etc Lower limb pain Pain and swelling of knee and surrounding tissues

Stomach Channel Points • Wei Jing Xue • 胃經穴

IDENTIFICATION	ACTION	INDICATIONS
ST-36 Zusanli 足三里 Foot Three Miles 3 CUN inferior to the lateral FORAMEN of the PATELLA (ST-35 Dubai), one finger breadth lateral to the anterior crest of the TIBIA. *He-SEA POINT* *EARTH POINT of the Stomach channel*	Tonifies Qi and Blood especially Stomach and Spleen Regulates Nutritive and Defensive Qi Expels Wind, Cold and Damp Raises Yang (use MOXA to ST-36 Zusanli with CV-6 Qihai and SV-20 Baihui) Regulates Intestines	Lack of vitality with weak muscle tone. Lack of appetite, epigastric pain and poor digestion Anaemia Sweating after Wind Cold invasion Fatigue of extremities Oedema Aching muscles and joints Knee problems Prolapse of organs especially Stomach and Intestines Abdominal distension and pain, constipation and diarrhoea
ST-40 Fenglong 豐隆 Abundant Bulge 8 CUN inferior to the lateral FORAMEN of the PATELLA (ST-35 Dubi), two finger breadths lateral to the anterior crest of the TIBIA. *Luo-CONNECTING POINT*	Resolves Damp and Phlegm Clears Stomach Heat Calms the Mind	Catarrh, phlegm as lumps/cysts Asthma, mental disturbances, muzzy or dizziness of the head Cloudy urine, mucus in stools Epigastric tightness and nervous anxiety Anxiety, fears and phobias due to lack of mental clarity
ST-42 Chongyang 重陽 Rushing Yang 1.3 SUN distal to ST-41 at the highest point of the DORSUM of the FOOT on the pulse of the DORSAL ARTERY *Yuan-SOURCE POINT*	Tonifies Stomach and Spleen Calms the Mind Removes Channel obstructions	Lack of appetite, epigastric pain and distension, constipation Anxiety Hysteria and chronic restlessness Weakness, pain, swelling and muscular wasting (atrophy) of the foot Coldness in all joints Paralysis of lower extremities

Stomach Channel Points • Wei Jing Xue • 胃經穴

IDENTIFICATION	ACTION	INDICATIONS
ST-44 Neiting 內廷 Inner Courtyard 0.5 CUN proximal to the dorsal web margin between the 2nd and 3rd TOES. *Ying-SPRING POINT* *WATER POINT of the Stomach channel*	Clears Heat Eliminates Wind from Face Stops pain Eliminates fullness	Bleeding gums, epigastric pain or burning sensation Heartburn Bleeding nose or gums Facial paralysis, trigeminal neuralgia Pain on stomach channel, particularly lower jaw, toothache Intestinal pain with fullness
ST-45 Lidui 厲兌 Strict Exchange About 0.1 CUN from the lateral corner of the 2nd TOENAIL, level with the base line of the nail. *Jing-WELL POINT* *METAL POINT of the Stomach channel*	Calms the Mind Clears Heat and Damp Heat	Insomnia, hysteria, disorientation and dream disturbed sleep Indigestion Facial oedema Toothache Sore throat Bleeding nose and gums

Spleen Channel Points • Pi Jing Xue • 脾經穴

IDENTIFICATION	ACTION	INDICATIONS
SP-1 Yinbai 隱白 Hidden White About 0.1 CUN from the medial corner of the 1st TOENAIL, level with the base line of the nail. *Jing-WELL POINT* *WOOD POINT of the Spleen channel*	Regulates Blood Strengthens the Spleen Calms the Mind	Stasis of blood in Uterus All types of bleeding due to Spleen deficiency including uterine, nasal, stomach, bladder or intestinal bleeding Excessive dreaming Depression and mental restlessness
SP-3 Taibai 太白 Supreme White Located proximal and inferior to the head of the 1st METATARSAL bone at the junction of the red and white skin. *Yuan-SOURCE POINT* *Shu-STREAM POINT* *EARTH POINT of the Spleen channel*	Strengthens the Spleen Resolves Damp Strengthens and straightens the Spine	Tiredness due to excessive mental work Lack of mental clarity and memory lapses Loose stools and diarrhoea Confused thinking, muzzy head, stuffy chest No appetite, epigastric fullness, abdominal bloating Difficult urination, cloudy urine and vaginal discharge Retention of phlegm in Lungs Chronic backache
SP-6 Sanyinjiao 三陰交 Three Yin Meeting Located 3 CUN directly superior to the vertex of the MEDIAL MALLEOLUS, on the posterior border of the TIBIA. *MEETING POINT of the Spleen, Liver and Kidney channels* **** Contra-indicated during pregnancy ****	Strengthens the Spleen Resolves Damp Smooths flow of Liver Qi Calms the Mind Tonifies Kidneys (Yin) Moves Blood Regulates Uterus and menstruation. Stops pain Promotes Labour	Loose stools and poor appetite Chronic tiredness (c/w ST-36 Zusanli) Mucus in stools, urinary infection or pain, vaginal discharge Painful menstruation Abdominal pain, constipation Irritability and frustration, insomnia Dry mouth with thirst Dizziness, tinnitus and night sweats Painful menstruation with clotted blood, dark blood in stools Any gynaecological complaint. Absence, excessive or painful menses, irregular menstrual cycle Delayed or difficult labour

Spleen Channel Points • Pi Jing Xue • 脾經穴

IDENTIFICATION	ACTION	INDICATIONS
SP-9 Yinlingquan 陰陵泉 Yin Mound Spring Located on the inferior border of the MEDIAL CONDYLE of the TIBIA in a depression between the posterior border of the TIBIA and the GASTROCNEMIUS muscle. *He-SEA POINT* *WATER POINT of the Spleen channel*	Resolves Dampness Benefits Lower Heater Removes Channel obstructions	Difficult urination, retention of urine, painful urination, cloudy urine Vaginal discharge Diarrhoea with foul smelling stools Oedema of the legs or abdomen Knee pain including swollen knee (Damp)
SP-10 Xuehai 血海 Sea of Blood With the KNEE flexed located 2 CUN superior to the medial superior ridge of the PATELLA on the VASTUS MEDIALIS muscle.	Removes stasis of Blood Cools the Blood	Acute or chronic, painful or irregular menstruation Psoriasis, eczema and skin rashes of hot nature Uterine bleeding between menses or excessive menstrual bleeding
SP-15 Daheng 大橫 Great Horizontal 4 CUN lateral to the centre of the umbilicus, directly below the nipple on the lateral border of the RECTUS ABDOMINUS muscle. *MEETING POINT of the Spleen channel with the Yin Tie vessel*	Strengthens the Spleen Strengthens the Limbs Resolves Damp Regulates Qi	Chronic constipation Cold and weak limbs Chronic diarrhoea with mucus in the stools Abdominal pain Sadness, weeping and sighing
SP-20 Zhourong 周榮 Surrounding Flourish 4 CUN lateral to the centre of the umbilicus, directly below the nipple on the lateral border of the RECTUS ABDOMINUS muscle. *MEETING POINT of the Spleen channel with the Yin Tie vessel*	Regulates Qi and unbinds the Chest	Pain and distension of the chest, costal and hypo-chondrial region Cough Coughing up phlegm Breathlessness
SP-21 Dabao 大包 Great Wrapper Located in the 6th INTERCOSTAL SPACE on the mid axillary line midway between the AXILLA (HT-1 Jiquan) and the free end of the 11th RIB (LV-13 Zhangmen). *GENERAL Luo-CONNECTING POINT of the Spleen*	Moves Blood in the blood connecting Channels	Muscular pain moving through the body due to blood stasis

Table 8.2 Functions of the Zang Fu (organ) and Zen Shiatsu (meridian) systems

ZANG FU 臟腑	SPLEEN organ Pi zang 脾臟	STOMACH organ Wei fu 胃腑
	Governs transformation and transportation	Controls reception, rotting and ripening of food and drink
	Controls the Blood (XUE)	Controls transportation of food essences
	Controls the Muscles and Limbs	Controls descending Qi
	Controls supportive Qi (maintains position of Organs)	Origin of Fluids
	Opens into Mouth	
	Manifests in the Lips	
	Houses Thought (YI)	
IMAGE	The **Official** who transforms and transports the grain	The **Official** who controls the grain storehouses where the five tastes derive
GOVERNMENT	**FINANCE MINISTER**	**TREASURY MINISTER**

ZEN SHIATSU 神指土	SPLEEN meridian Pi jing 脾經	STOMACH meridian Wei jing 胃經
	Governs secretion of digestive enzymes	Governs the upper digestive tract through lips, oesophagus, stomach, and duodenum to the jejunum
	Reproductive hormones in relation to mammaries, ovaries, testes and uterus	Controls appetite, lactation, ovarian, testicular and uterine function
	Promotes mental clarity	
BASIC	Transforms and Transports Ki via Food and the Intellect	Receives Ki via Food and Drink
SPECIFIC	**FOOD & INTELLECTUAL DIGESTION**	**INTAKE OF FOOD KI**
GENERAL	**NOURISHMENT**	

Table 8.3 Zen Shiatsu correspondences: Stomach meridian

STOMACH meridian		Weijing 胃經
FACULTY	Spiritual Input	: Yi, via Spleen meridian
	Functions via	: Intelligence
	Represents	: Nurturing
	Supplemented by	: Intake of Food & Emotive Ki
	Realised by	: Fulfilling
	Dominant Zone	: Front
	Embryological Layer	: Mesoderm
	Meridian Nature	: Yang
	Tuning Time	: 7am - 9am
ANATOMY & PHYSIOLOGY	Eyes	] Appetite Mechanism
	Mouth	] Digestive System
	Oesophagus	]
	Stomach	]
	Pyloric Sphincter	]
	Duodenum	]
	Jejunum	]
	Mammaries	] Hormonal System
	Ovaries, Testes	] Reproductive System
	Uterus	] Menstrual Cycle
PHYSICAL	Anaemia	Lactation Problems
	Appetite Disorders	Menstrual Cycle Disorders
	Belching	Nasal Problems
	Cold Sores	Poor Circulation- Lower Limbs
	Coldness in Digestive System	Ptosis - Visceral (Stomach)
	Colds & Flu	Pyrosis (Heartburn)
	Dry Complexion	Shoulder Pain
	Epigastric Discomfort	Stomach Problems/Ulcers
	Eye Problems	Thirst
	Halitosis (Bad Breath)	Toothache
PSYCHOLOGICAL	Affection	Maternal Issues
	Anxiety	Moody
	Burdened	Neurotic
	Compensatory Eating	Overactive
	Family (Relationships)	Overeating
	Frustration	Overthinking
	Future Orientated	Satisfaction
	Gullibility	Searching
	Hashing over Things	Stubborn
	Love	Unreliable

STOMACH meridian   Weijing 胃經

Table 8.4 Zen Shiatsu correspondences: Spleen meridian

SPLEEN meridian		Pi jing 脾經
FACULTY	Spiritual Input	: Yi, Thought
	Functions via	: Intelligence
	Represents	: Fertility
	Supplemented by	: Food & Intellectual Digestion
	Realised by	: Creating
	Dominant Zone	: Front
	Embryological Layer	: Mesoderm
	Meridian Nature	: Yin
	Tuning Time	: 9am - 11am
ANATOMY & PHYSIOLOGY	Cerebral Cortex	] Mento-Sensory Initiative
	Cerebrum	] Muscular System
	Muscles	]
	Lips	] Taste Mechanism
	Tongue	] Digestive System/
	Salivary Glands	] Enzymes
	Pancreas	]
	Gall Bladder	]
	Jejunum	]
	Mammaries	] Hormonal System
	Ovaries,Testes	] Reproductive System
	Uterus	] Menstrual Cycle
PHYSICAL	Anaemia	Knee/Muscle Problems
	Appetite Disorders	Lack of Exercise
	Biliousness	Lack of Saliva
	Blood Disorders	Loose Stools
	Brownish Face	Memory Problems
	Craving Food/Liquids	Menstrual/Fertility problems
	Digestive Disorders	Navel Stiffness
	Diabetes	Spinal Pain (Lower)
	Headaches	Sticky Dry Taste
	Heaviness in Limbs	Weight Problems
PSYCHOLOGICAL	Anguish	Overtechnical
	Anxiety	Overthinking
	Attention Seeking	Receptiveness
	Confidence	Restlessness
	Drowsy/Sleepiness	Self Pity
	Eating Habits	Stubborn
	Expressiveness	Support
	Home Life Issues (Family)	Timidity
	Intellectualisation	Worry
	Nervousness	Yearning (Maternal)

Fig. 8.2 Anterior upper view: Zen Shiatsu Stomach and Spleen meridians

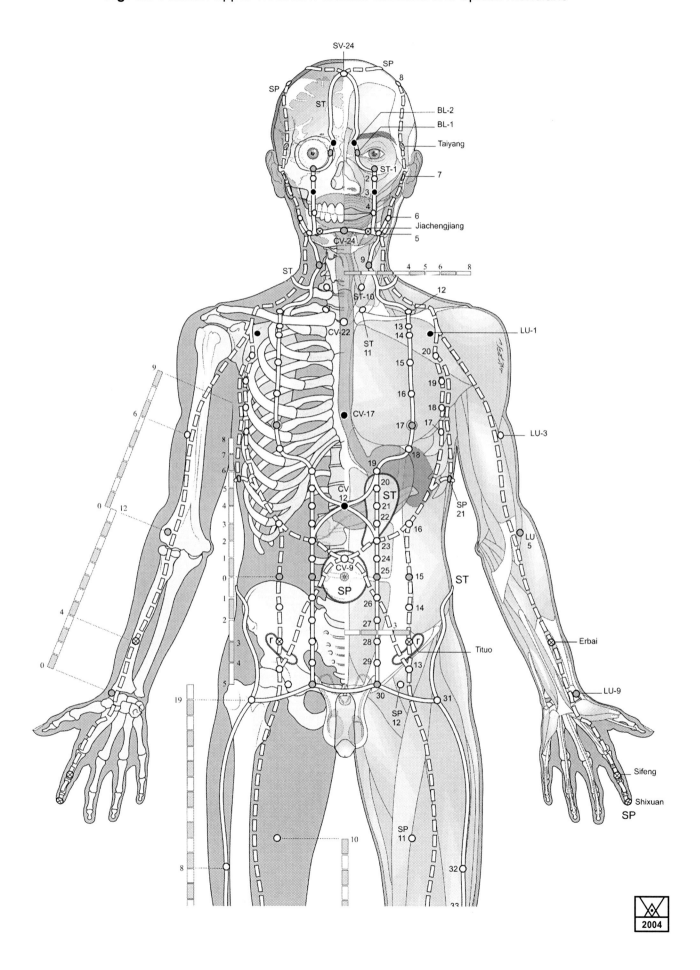

Fig. 8.3 Anterior lower view: Zen Shiatsu Stomach and Spleen meridians

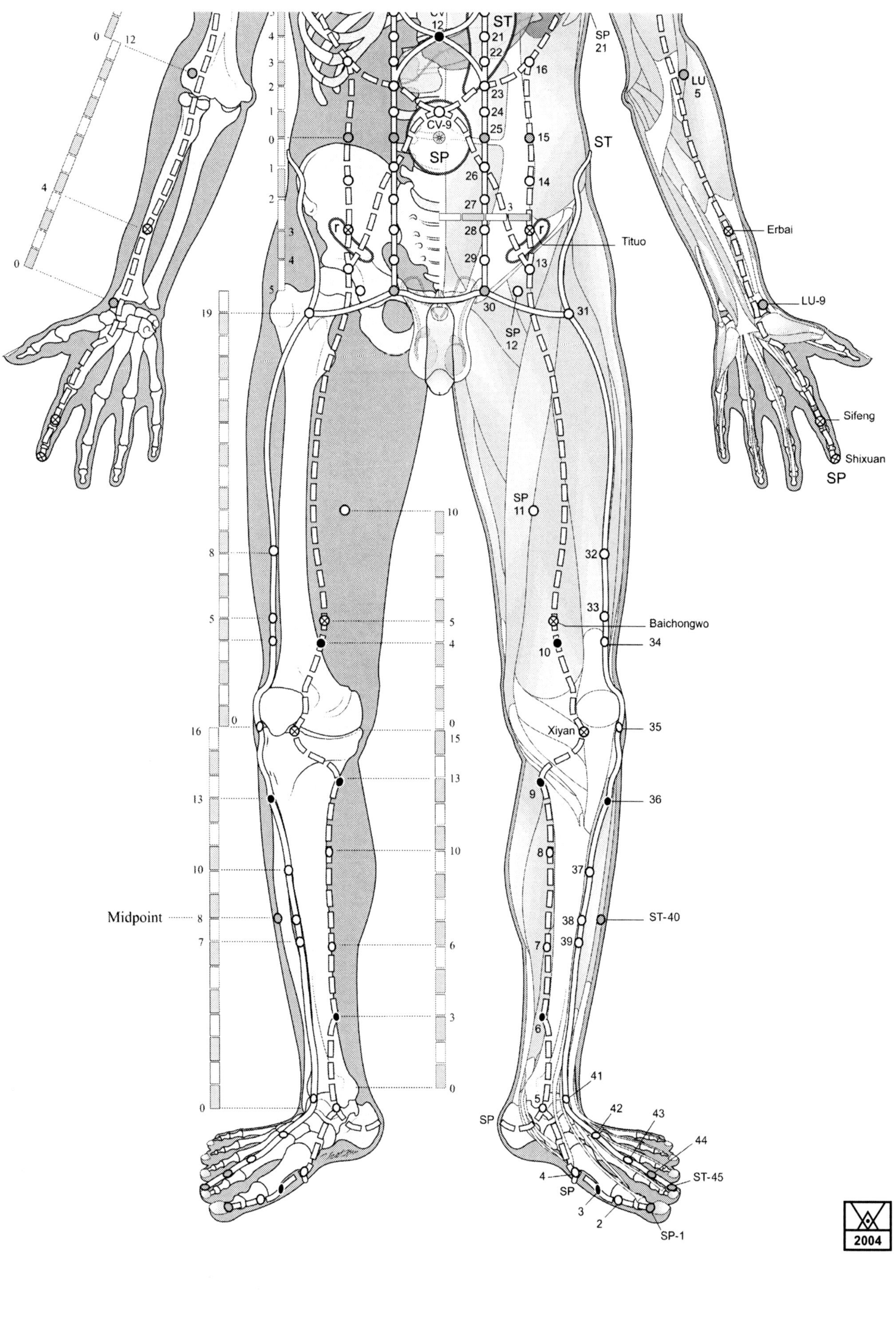

Fig. 8.4 Posterior upper view: Zen Shiatsu Stomach and Spleen meridians

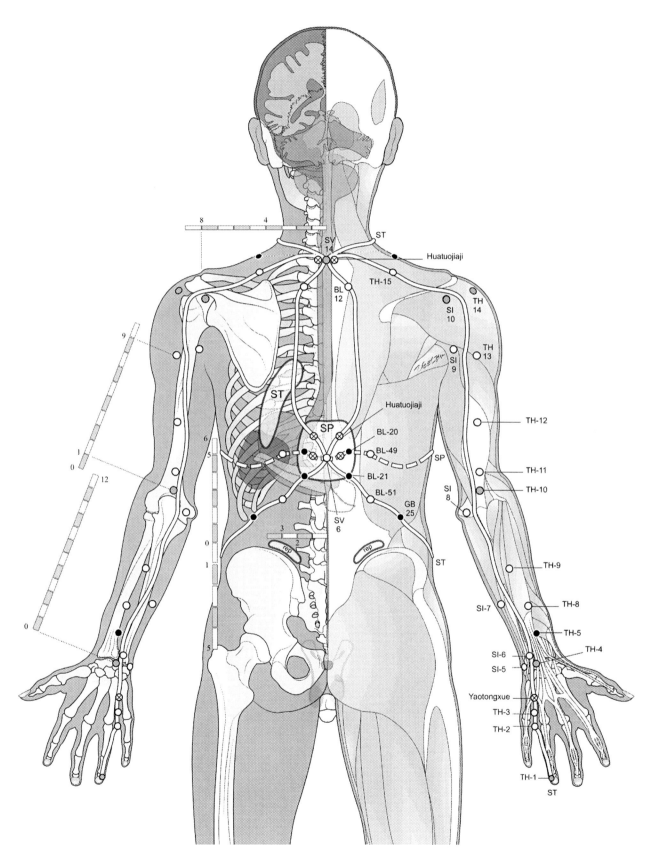

Fig. 8.5 Posterior lower view: Zen Shiatsu Stomach and Spleen meridians

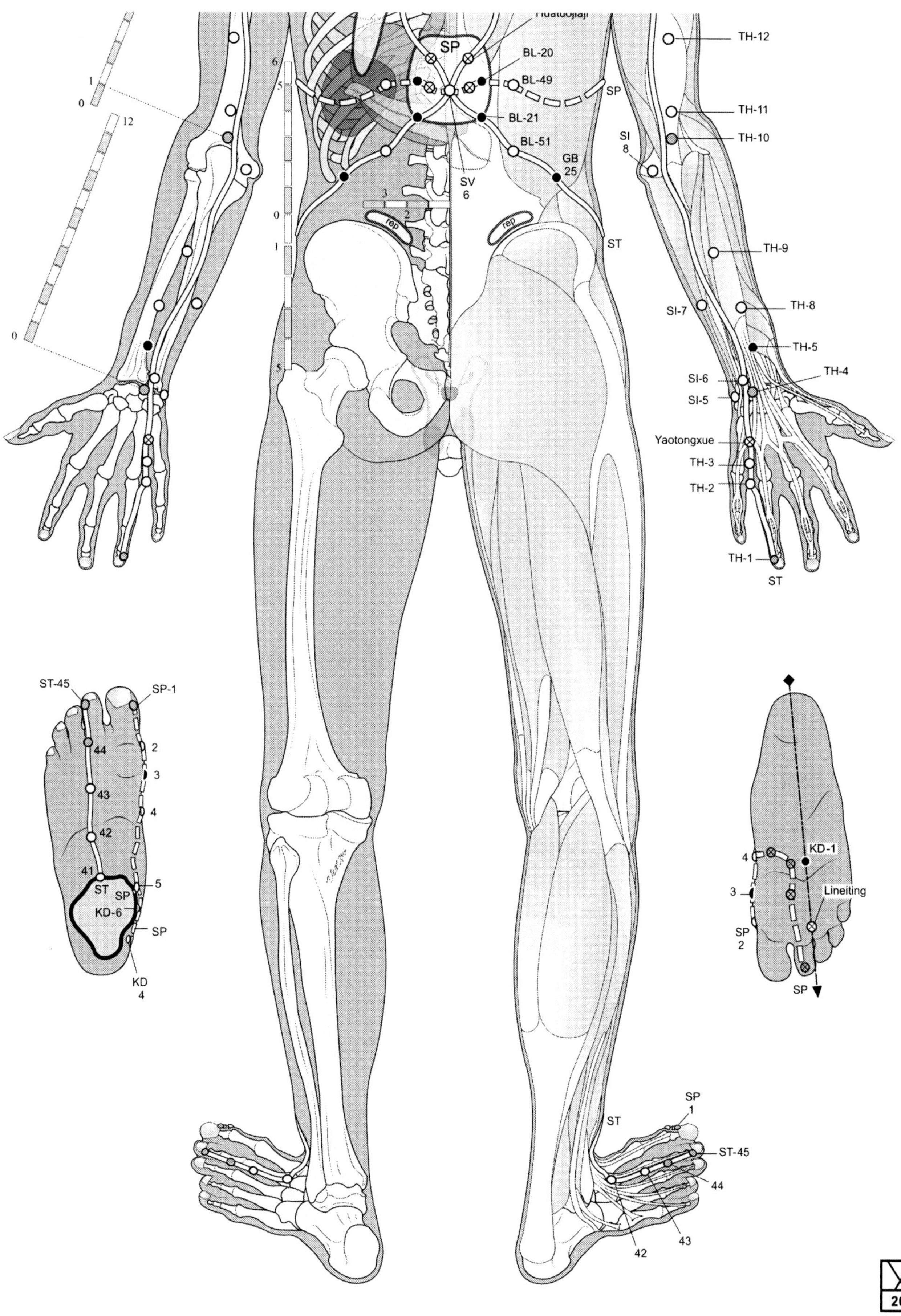

Huatuojiaji
SP
BL-20
BL-49
SP
BL-21
BL-51
SV
6
GB
25
ST
SI
8
TH-12
TH-11
TH-10
TH-9
TH-8
SI-7
TH-5
SI-6
TH-4
SI-5
Yaotongxue
TH-3
TH-2
TH-1
ST
rep
rep

ST-45
SP-1
44
2
3
43
4
42
41
5
ST
SP
KD-6
SP
KD
4

4
KD-1
3
Lineiting
SP
2
SP

SP
1
ST
ST-45
44
43
42

Fig. 8.6 Head cranial and lateral details: Zen Shiatsu Stomach and Spleen meridians

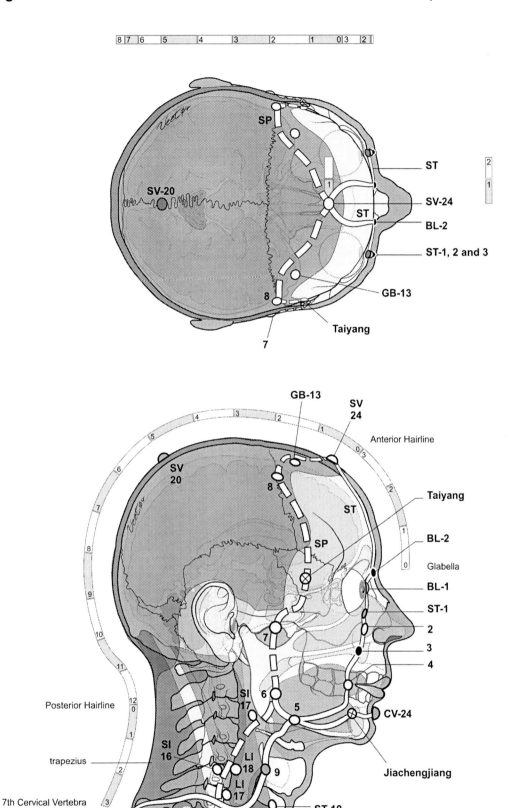

Fig. 8.7 Lower arm and hand: Zen Shiatsu Stomach and Spleen channels

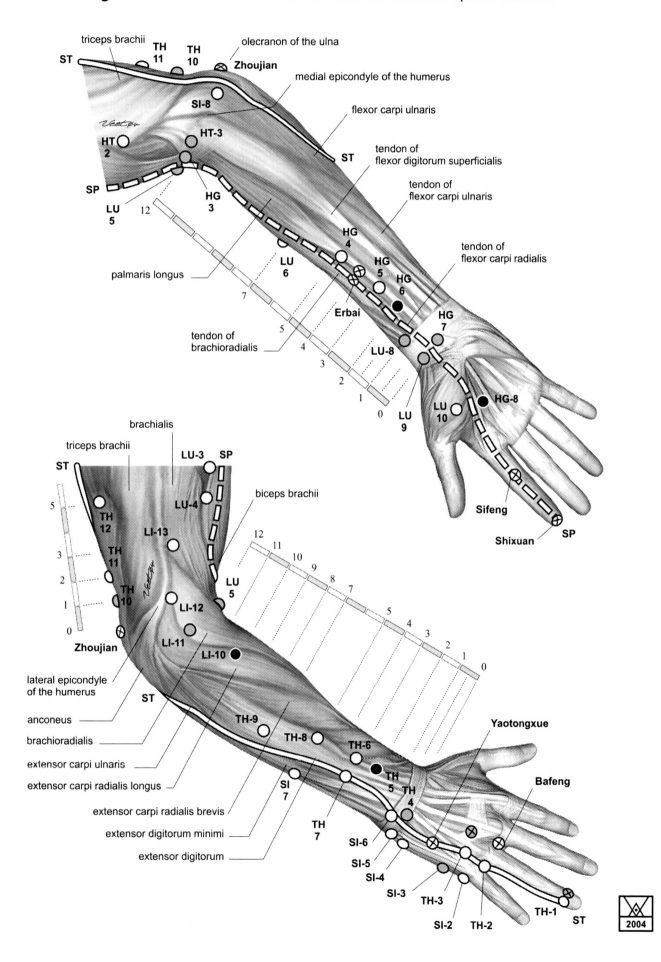

Fig. 8.8 Lower Leg and Foot details: Zen Shiatsu Stomach and Spleen meridians

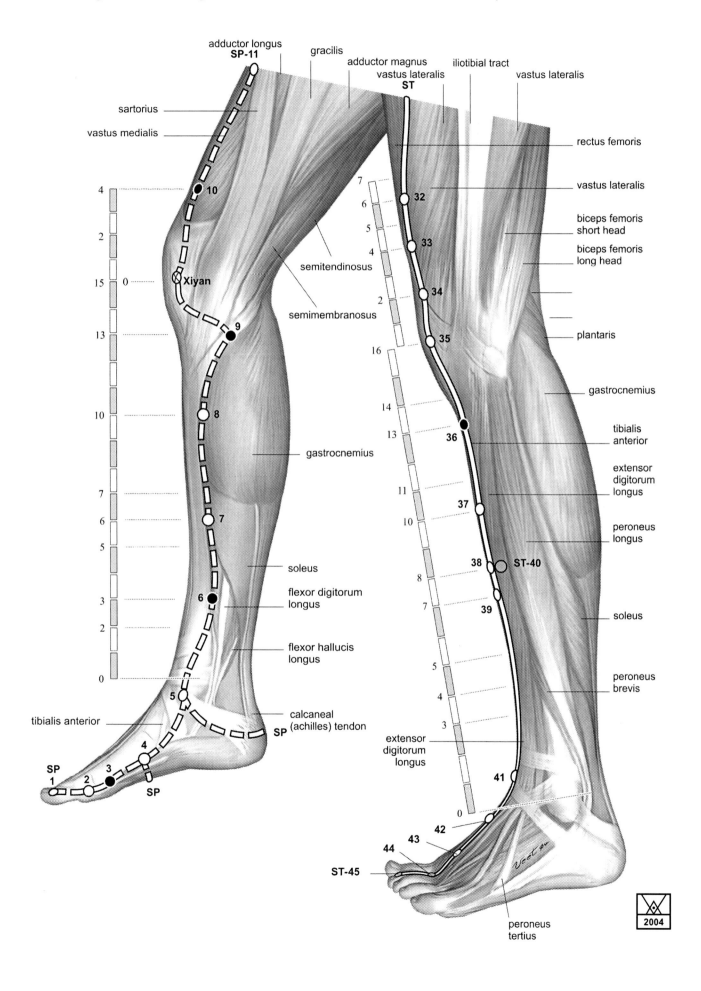

Fig. 8.9 Foot dorsal and plantar details: Zen Shiatsu Stomach and Spleen meridians

Foot: Dorsal view

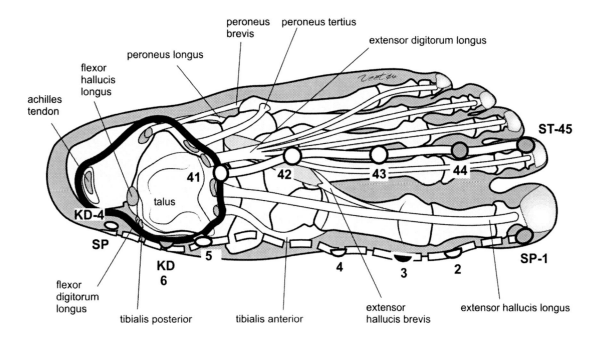

Foot: Plantar view

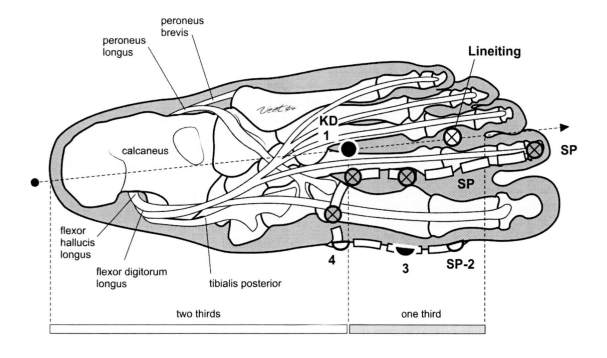

Chapter 9
the METAL element

Lung
and
Large Intestine

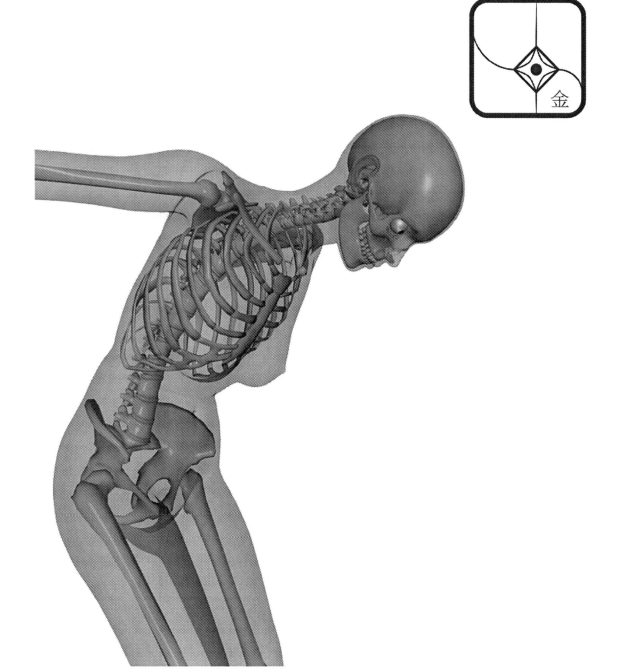

Fig. 9.1 The Five element sequences: METAL

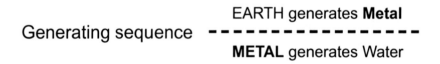

Fire

Wood

Earth

Water

METAL

Generating sequence

EARTH generates **Metal**

- - - - - - - - - - - - - - - - - -

METAL generates Water

Control sequence

FIRE controls **Metal**

————————————

METAL controls Wood

Table 9.1 The Five element correspondences: METAL

The METAL element		Jin xing 金行
FACULTY	Spiritual	: Po, Corporeal Soul Vitality
	Celestial Stems	: Geng (stem 7) Xin (stem 8)
	Earthly branches	: Shen (branch 9) and You (branch 10)
	Planet	: Venus
	Number	: 9
	Pentatonic note	: Shang, (Ray, 2nd note of scale)
	Genetic aspiration	: Interaction via communication
	Cycle	: Harvest
	Yin/Yang	: Lesser Yin
	Quality	: Solidified
ENVIRONMENTAL	Season	: Autumn
	Phase of Moon	: Half moon decreasing to new moon
	Climate	: Dry
	Direction	: West
	Colour	: White
	Part of the Day	: Evening
BODY	Organ Yin	: Lung
	Yang	: Large Intestine
	Tissue	: Skin
	Skin Colour	: White, Pale
	Odour	: Rotten
	Branch	: Body Hair
	Sense Organ	: Nose
	Senses	: Smell
	Fluid	: Mucus
EMOTIONAL	Emotion	: Grief, Positivity
	Sound, Voice	: Weeping, Wailing
	Action	: Coughing
FOOD (symbol)	Animal	: Horse
	Taste	: Spicy
	Fruit	: Peach
	Grain	: Rice
	Vegetable	: Small and contracted (ginger, onion, radish)

Lung Channel Points • Fei Jing Xue • 肺經穴

IDENTIFICATION	ACTION	INDICATIONS
LU-1 Zhongfu 中府 Middle Palace 1 CUN inferior to the centre of the INFRACLAVICULAR FOSSA and 6 CUN lateral to the Controller vessel. *FRONT Mu-COLLECTING POINT of the Lung* *MEETING POINT of the Lung and Spleen channels*	Regulates Lung Qi Stops Cough Clears Heat Stimulates descending of Lung Qi Fullness of Chest Stops pain	Asthma Bronchitis with cough and wheezing Breathing difficulties Painful throat Stagnation from phlegm or blood stasis Shoulder or upper back pain
LU-5 Chize 尺澤 Cubit Marsh With ELBOW slightly flexed, located on the transverse CUBITAL crease on the RADIAL side of the TENDON of the BICEPS BRACHII muscle. *He-SEA POINT* *WATER POINT of the Lung channel* **** Use Moxibustion with caution ****	Clears Lung Heat Expels Phlegm (Hot and Cold) Relaxes Sinew	Asthma Bronchitis Cough, fever, thirst and yellow sputum Yellow or white sputum Chilliness Pain and swelling of elbow and arm Inability to raise arm to head
LU-7 Leique 列缺 Broken Sequence 1.5 CUN above the transverse crease of the WRIST. Proximal to the STYLOID process of the RADIUS. *Luo-CONNECTING POINT* *OPENING POINT of the Controller vessel* *Ma Dan-yang HEAVENLY STAR POINT*	Stimulates descending and dispersal of Lung Qi Expels Exterior Wind (Cold/Hot) Opens Nose Benefits Bladder and Water Passages Assists Emotional Expression Balances the Po (corporeal soul)	Asthma, cough Common cold, flu, stiff neck, headache Sinus problems Sneezing, runny nose and loss of sense of smell Oedema and urinary retention Suppression of feelings related to worry, grief, sadness etc Tense shoulders with shallow breathing

Lung Channel Points • Fei Jing Xue • 肺經穴

IDENTIFICATION	ACTION	INDICATIONS
LU-9 Taiyuan 太淵 Supreme Abyss Located on the transverse crease of the WRIST, at the RADIAL side of the RADIAL ARTERY between the RADIUS and the SCAPHOID bones. *Yuan-SOURCE POINT* *Shu-STREAM POINT* *EARTH POINT of the Lung channel* *Hui-MEETING POINT of the BLOOD VESSELS*	Tonifies Lung Qi and gathering Qi Resolves Phlegm Promotes Blood circulation Tonifies Heart Qi	Lack of vitality Chronic tiredness Cold hands with weak voice Dry cough Chronic cough with yellow sticky sputum Poor circulation Cold hands and feet Chilblains and varicose veins Breathless on exertion Palpitations
LU-11 Shaoshang 少商 Lesser (Metal's) Tone Located about 0.1 CUN from the RADIAL corner of the THUMBNAIL, level with the base line of the nail. *Jing-WELL POINT* *WOOD POINT of the Lung channel* *Sun Si Mao GHOST POINT*	Expels External and Interior Wind Promotes resuscitation	Sore throat Dry mouth High fever with sweating Loss of consciousness

Large Intestine Channel Points • Da Chang Jing Xue • 大腸經穴

IDENTIFICATION	ACTION	INDICATIONS
LI-1 Shangyang 商陽 (Metal's) Tone Yang Located about 0.1 CUN from the RADIAL corner of the 2nd FINGERNAIL, level with the base line of the nail. *Jing-WELL POINT* *METAL POINT of the Large Intestine channel*	Clears Heat Expels Wind and Cold Removes obstructions Revives consciousness	Sore throat Acute conjunctivitis Shoulder pain radiating to the Supraclavicular Fossa Loss of consciousness
LI-4 Hegu 合谷 Joining Valley On the dorsum of the HAND, at the web and groove between the 1st and 2nd METACARPAL bones, level with the midpoint of the 2nd METACARPAL bone and near its RADIAL border. *Yuan-SOURCE POINT* *Ma Dan-yang HEAVENLY STAR POINT* **** Contra-indicated during pregnancy ****	Expels Wind Heat Releases the Exterior Promotes descending of Lung Qi Stops pain Removes Channel obstructions Calms the Mind (roots Qi to *Hara*) Strengthens defensive Qi Promotes Labour	Nasal congestion, sneezing, burning eyes, hay fever Cough, stiff neck, aversion to cold Common cold and flu Intestinal and uterine pain Arm or shoulder pain, toothache, frontal headache, sinusitis, trigeminal neuralgia, facial paralysis Anxiety Asthma, bronchitis, cold etc Delayed or difficult labour
LI-10 Shousanli 手三里 Arm Three Miles Located on the RADIAL side of the forearm, 2 CUN distal to LI-11 Quchi, on a line connecting to LI-5 Yangxi (at the RADIAL side of the wrist).	Removes Channel obstructions Tonifies Qi	Any muscular problem affecting the arm and hands Wasting of arm muscles Sluggish intestines Lack of vitality (especially upper body)

Large Intestine Channel Points • Da Chang Jing Xue • 大腸經穴

IDENTIFICATION	ACTION	INDICATIONS
LI-11 Quchi 曲池 Pool at the Crook With the ELBOW flexed, located between the lateral end of the transverse CUBITAL crease and the LATERAL EPICONDYLE of the HUMERUS. *He-SEA POINT* *EARTH POINT of the Large Intestine channel* *Ma Dan-yang HEAVENLY STAR POINT*	Expels Exterior Wind Clears Heat Cools Blood Clears Damp Heat Removes Channel obstructions Benefits the Sinews	Fever, chills, stiff neck, sweating, runny nose and body aches Eczema, psoriasis, urticaria (nettle rash) Skin eruptions (acne) Cystitis and urethritis Heavy feeling, loose stools, abdominal distension Goitre (thyroid swelling) Muscular wasting (atrophy) Pain and paralysis of arm and shoulders Rheumatism and arthritis
LI-15 Jianyu 肩髃 Shoulder's Corner Located directly inferior to the anterior border of the ACROMION where a depression is formed when the ARM is abducted.	Removes Channel obstructions Benefits Sinews Stops Shoulder pain Expels Wind and clears Heat	Frozen shoulder Shoulder bursitis (inflammation), pain or stiffness Atrophy (wasting) of upper limbs Muscular spasms Paralysis of arm Urticaria (nettle rash) due to Wind-Heat Excessive sweating
LI-16 Jugu 巨骨 Great Bone Located in the depression between the ACROMION extremity of the CLAVICLE and the SCAPULAR SPINE.	Removes Channel obstructions Opens Chest Stimulates descending of Lung Qi Subdues ascending rebellious Qi	Frozen shoulder Inflammation, pain and stiffness of shoulder and upper back zone Asthma, Breathlessness and cough Hypertension
LI-20 Yingxiang 迎香 Welcome Fragrance Located on the NASOLABIAL SULCUS, level with the mid point of the lateral border of the ALA NASI.	Dispels Exterior Wind	All nose problems Sneezing Loss of sense of smell Bleeding nose, runny nose, stuffy nose, Allergic rhinitis (nasal inflammation) Sinusitis

Table 9.2 Functions of the Zang Fu (organ) and Zen Shiatsu (meridian) systems

ZANG FU 臟腑	LUNG organ Fei zang 肺臟	LARGE INTESTINE organ Da Chang fu 大腸腑
	Governs Qi and Respiration Controls dispersing and descending Controls Channels and Blood Vessels Regulates Water Passages Controls Skin and Body Hair Opens into Nose Houses Corporeal Soul (PO)	Receives impure Material, absorbs Liquid and excretes the Stools
IMAGE	The **Minister** from whom policies are derived	The **Official** in charge of transmission
GOVERNMENT	**PRIME MINISTER**	**FOREIGN MINISTER**

ZEN SHIATSU 神指土	LUNG meridian Fei jing 肺經	LARGE INTESTINE meridian Da Chang jing 大腸經
	Governs Respiration via intake of Ki and elimination of Gases by exhalation Relates to regulation of Brain function and state of Mind	Elimination and excretion of waste material Harmonise emotions via appropriate hold on/let go response
BASIC	Exchange of Gases via Respiration for Survival	Elimination of Processed Food and Emotive Ki
SPECIFIC	**INTAKE OF PURE KI**	**ELIMINATION**
GENERAL	**VITALITY**	

Table 9.3 Zen Shiatsu correspondences: Lung meridian

LUNG meridian			Fei jing 肺經
FACULTY	Spiritual Input	:	Po, Corporeal Soul
	Functions via	:	Physical Body
	Represents	:	Structure
	Supplemented by	:	Intake of Pure Ki
	Realised by	:	Interacting
	Dominant Zone	:	Outside
	Embryological Layer	:	Ectoderm
	Meridian Nature	:	Yin
	Tuning Time	:	3am - 5am
ANATOMY & PHYSIOLOGY	Medulla Oblongata, Pons	]	Respiratory Rythmic Centre
	Nose	]	Respiratory System
	Sinuses	]	
	Pharynx	]	Vocals
	Larynx	]	
	Bronchi	]	Related to Brain Functioning
	Lungs	]	
	Intercostal Muscles	]	
	Diaphragm	]	
	Skin (Pores)	]	Integumentary System
PHYSICAL	Asthma		Fever
	Bronchitis		Headaches
	Colds & Flu		Heavy Headiness
	Congestion of Nose/Chest		Loss of Voice
	Constipation		Pale Complexion
	Coughs		Respiratory Disease
	Dizziness		Stiff Thumb
	Dry Skin		Tight Intercostal Muscles
	Emphysema		Upper Back Pain
	Extreme Fatigue		White of Eyes, Dull
PSYCHOLOGICAL	Crying/Weeping		Pent Up Emotions
	Depression		Reclusive
	Hypersensitivity		Rigid Concepts
	Inability to Relax		Selfishness
	Jealousy		Shallow Breathing
	Lack of Clear Thinking		Sighing
	Melancholy		Social Problems
	Obsessed with Details		Unending Grief
	Organisational Problems		Unenthusiastic
	Overanxious		Worry
LUNG meridian			Fei jing 肺經

Table 9.4 Zen Shiatsu correspondences: Large Intestine meridian

LARGE INTESTINE meridian		Da Chang jing 大腸經
FACULTY	Spiritual Input	: Po, via Lung meridian
	Functions via	: Physical Body
	Represents	: Borders
	Supplemented by	: Elimination
	Realised by	: Clarifying
	Dominant Zone	: Outside
	Embryological Layer	: Ectoderm
	Meridian Nature	: Yang
	Tuning Time	: 5am - 7am
ANATOMY & PHYSIOLOGY	Nose	] Respiratory System
	Sinuses	]
	Mouth	] Digestive System
	Ileocaecal Valve	] Mucus Excretions
	Large Intestine	] Bowel Movement
	Anal (Internal and External)	]
	Sphincters	]
	Skin	] Integumentary System
PHYSICAL	Coldness in Lower Hara	Intestinal Disease
	Colds & Flu	Jaw Problems
	Constipation	Nasal Congestion
	Diarrhoea	Oedema
	Dislike of Exercise	Shoulder Pain
	Dull Vision	Skin Problems
	Epistaxis (Nose Bleeds)	Tonsillitis
	Haemorrhoids	Toothache
	Headaches	Stiff Index Finger
	Hip Problems	Stiffness in general
PSYCHOLOGICAL	Casualness	Overbearing Attitude
	Closed Off	Overdependence
	Easily Disappointed	Relationship Difficulties
	Holding on/Hoarding	Releasing/Letting Go
	Insecurity	Rigidity
	Lack of Expression	Social Problems
	Laziness	Stuckness
	No Enthusiasm	Territorial Issues
	No Initiative	Unhappiness
	Opinionated	Worthiness

Fig. 9.2 Anterior upper view: Zen Shiatsu Lung and Large Intestine meridians

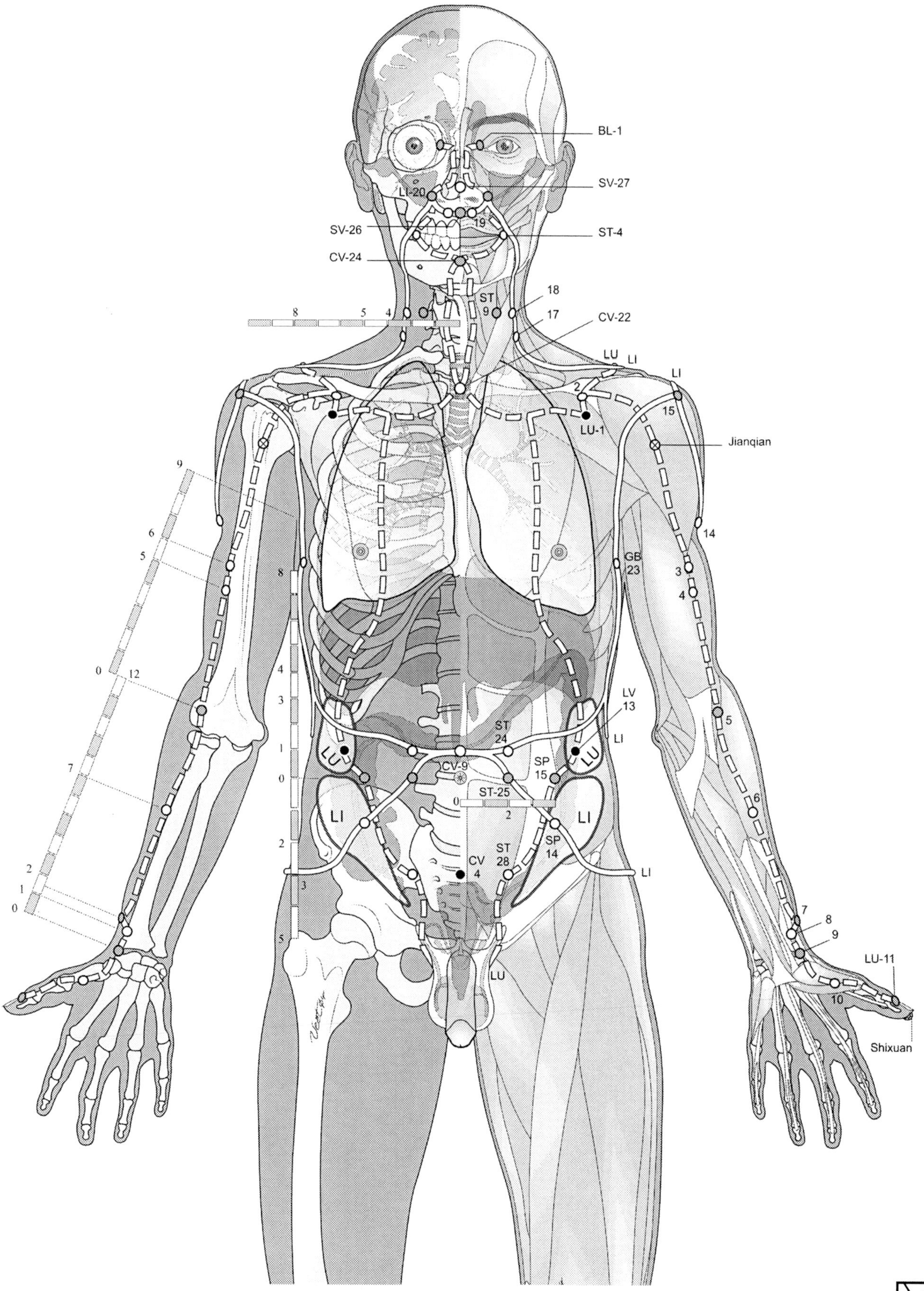

Fig. 9.3 Posterior upper view: Zen Shiatsu Lung and Large Intestine meridians

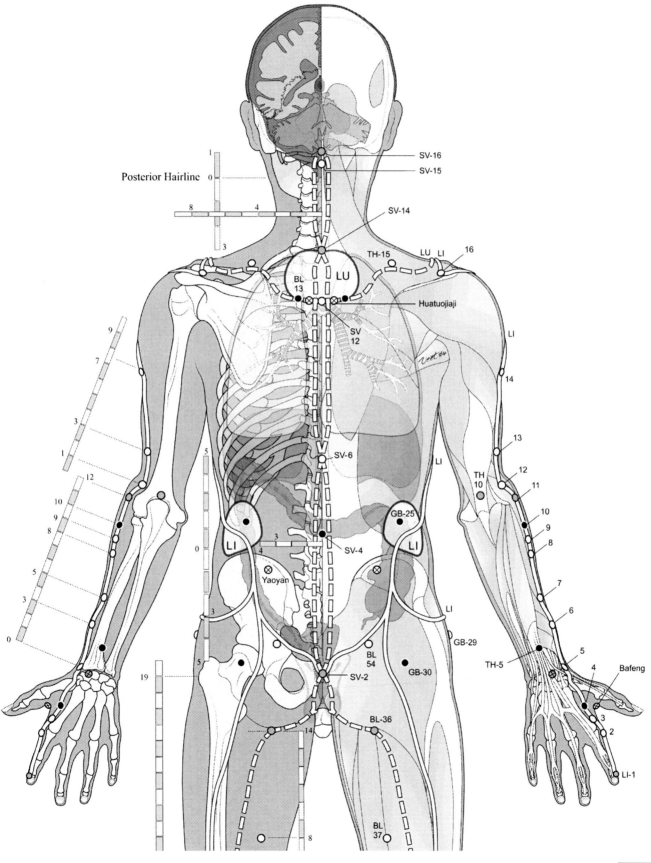

Fig. 9.4 Posterior lower view: Zen Shiatsu Lung and Large Intestine meridians

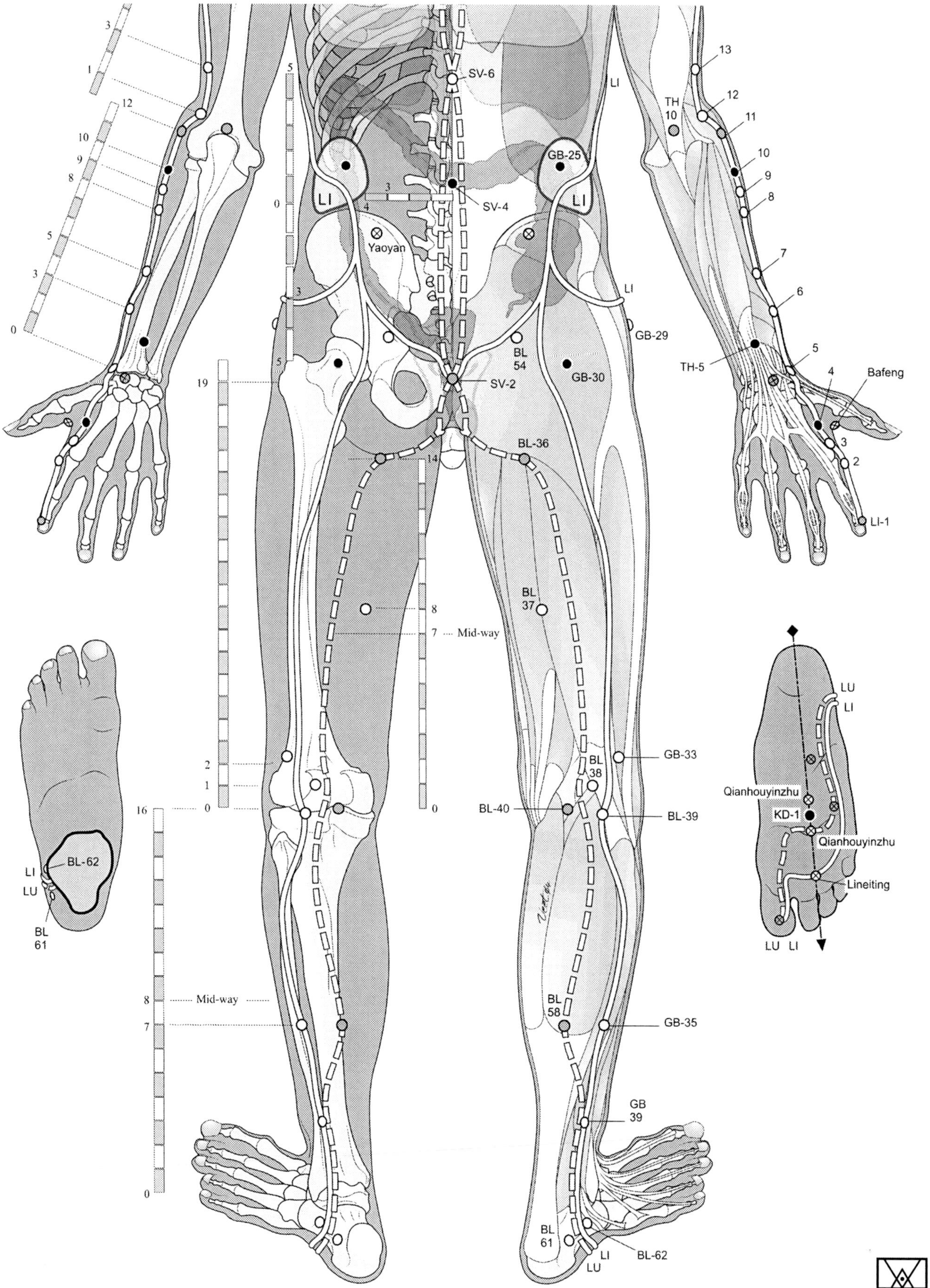

Fig. 9.5 Head cranial and lateral details: Zen Shiatsu Lung and Large Intestine meridians

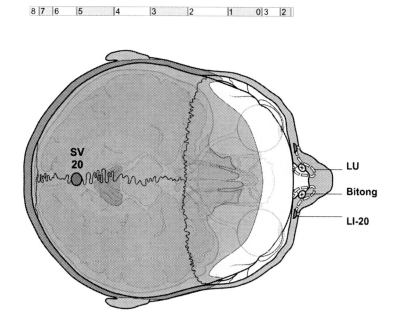

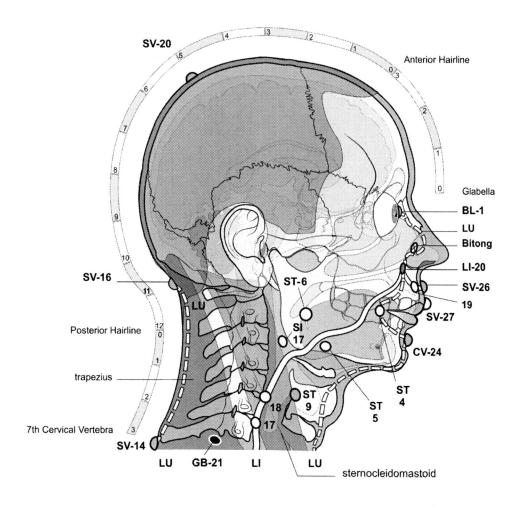

Fig. 9.6 Lower arm and hand: Zen Shiatsu Lung and Large Intestine channels

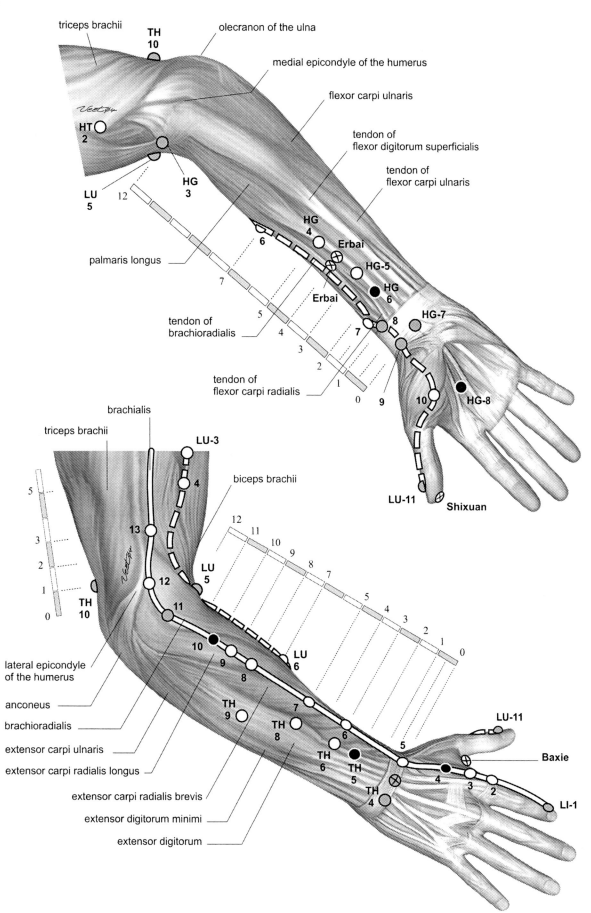

Fig. 9.7 Male Perineum details: Zen Shiatsu Lung and Large Intestine meridians

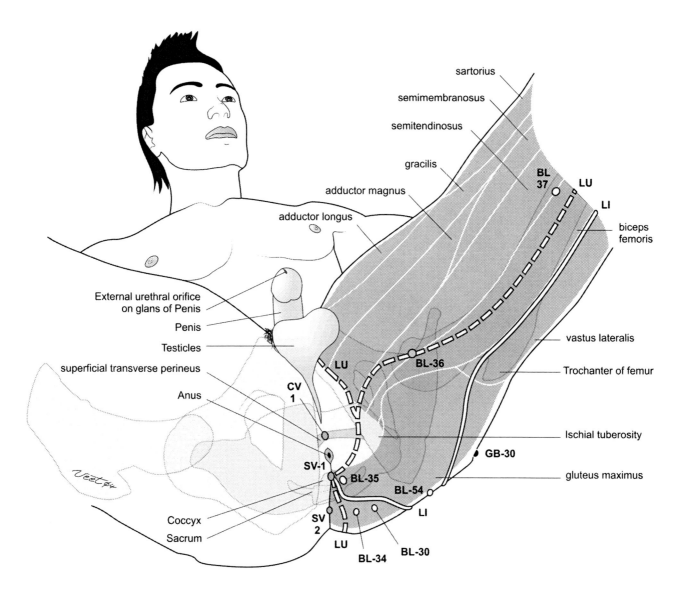

Fig. 9.8 Female Perineum details: Zen Shiatsu Lung and Large Intestine meridians

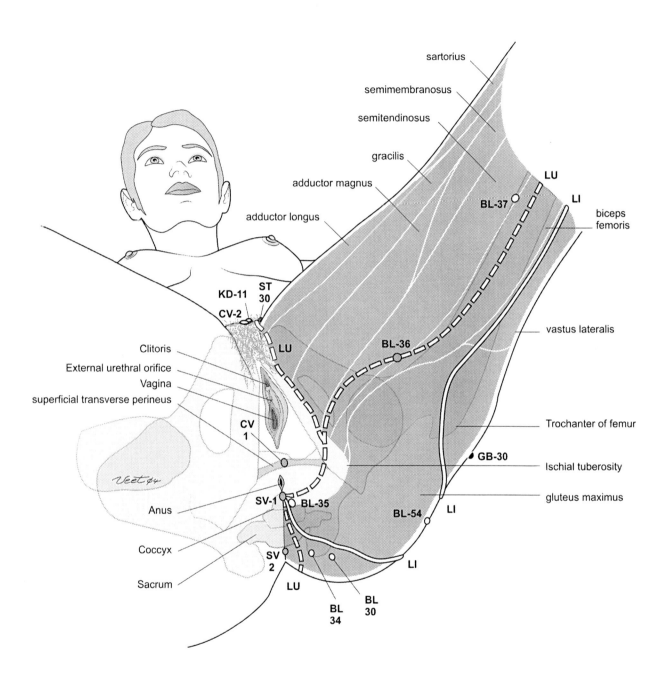

Fig. 9.9 Lower Leg and Foot details: Zen Shiatsu Lung and Large Intestine meridians

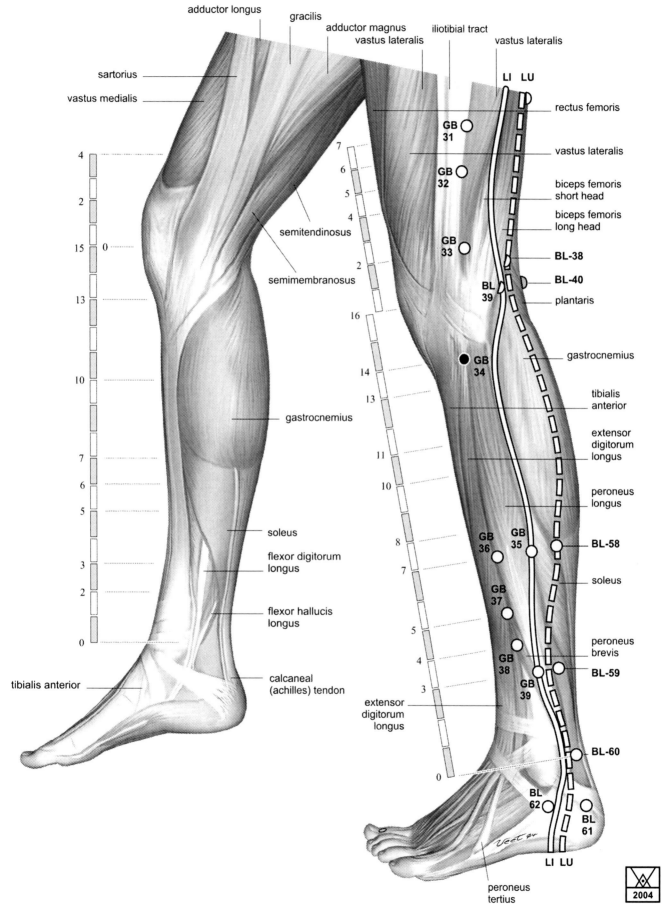

Fig. 9.10 Foot dorsal and plantar details: Zen Shiatsu Lung and Large Intestine meridians

Foot: Dorsal view

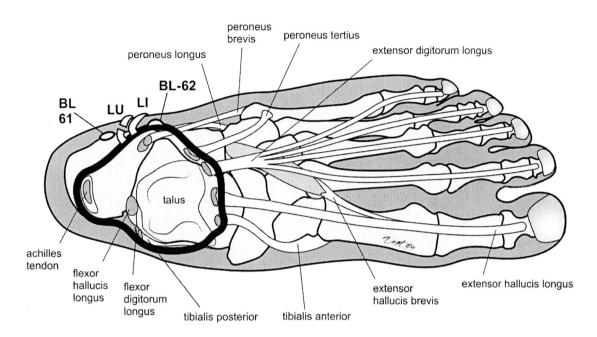

peroneus
brevis
peroneus longus   peroneus tertius
                                    extensor digitorum longus

BL-62

**BL
61**   **LU** **LI**

talus

achilles
tendon
flexor
hallucis   flexor
longus   digitorum
longus   tibialis posterior   tibialis anterior
                    extensor
                    hallucis brevis   extensor hallucis longus

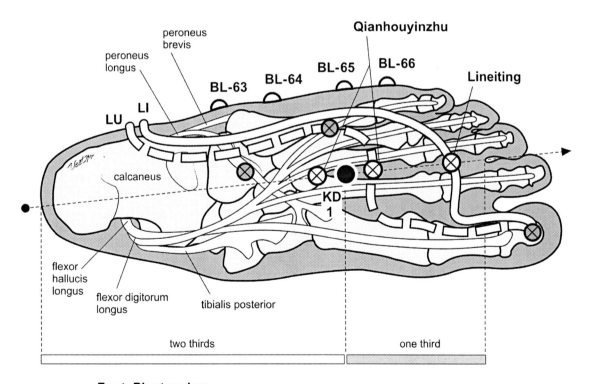

Qianhouyinzhu

peroneus
brevis
peroneus
longus   **BL-65** **BL-66**
LU LI   **BL-63** **BL-64**   **Lineiting**

calcaneus

KD
1

flexor
hallucis
longus
flexor digitorum
longus   tibialis posterior

two thirds   one third

Foot: Plantar view

Chapter 10
COMPOSITE illustrations
Zen Shiatsu composites
with
Anatomical cross sections

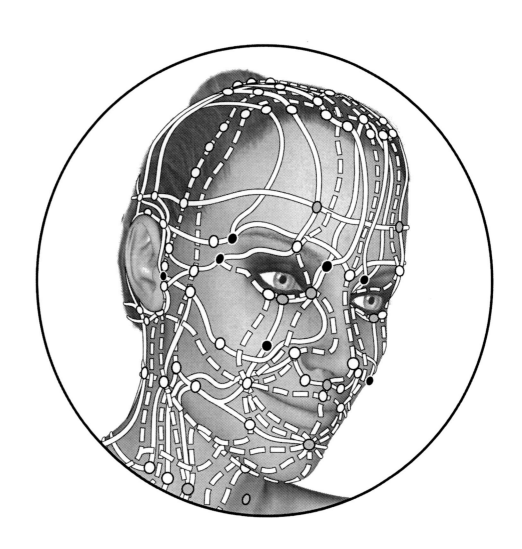

Fig. 10.1 Anterior upper view: Zen Shiatsu meridians

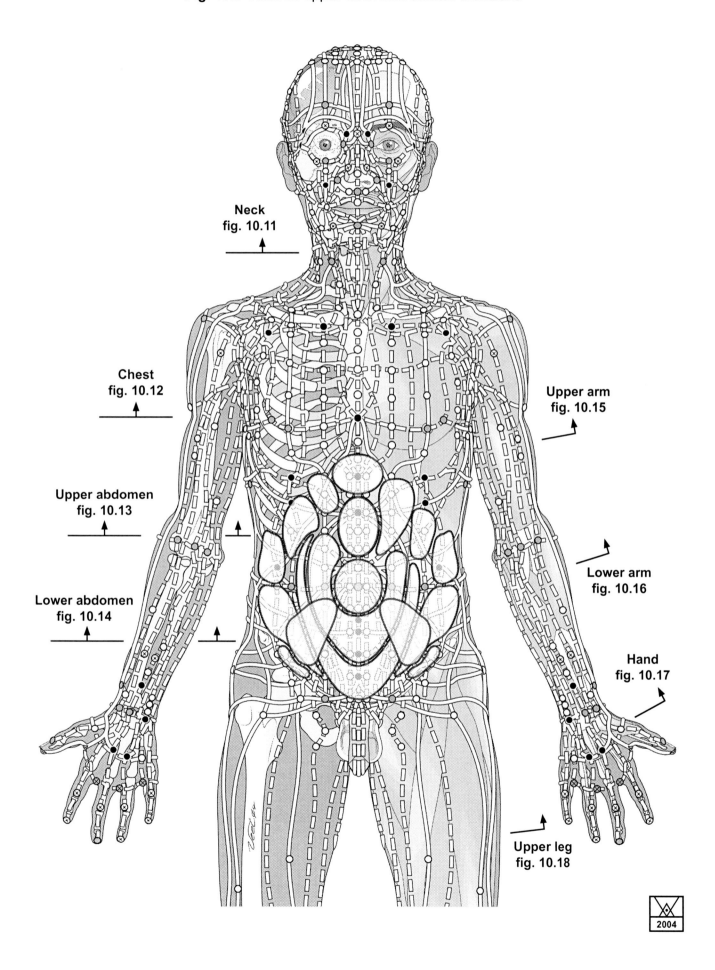

Neck
fig. 10.11

Chest
fig. 10.12

Upper abdomen
fig. 10.13

Lower abdomen
fig. 10.14

Upper arm
fig. 10.15

Lower arm
fig. 10.16

Hand
fig. 10.17

Upper leg
fig. 10.18

2004

Fig. 10.2 Anterior lower view: Zen Shiatsu meridians

Upper abdomen
fig. 10.13

Lower abdomen
fig. 10.14

Lower arm
fig. 10.16

Hand
fig. 10.17

Upper leg
fig. 10.18

Lower leg
fig. 10.19

fig. 10.20

2004

Fig. 10.3 Posterior upper view: Zen Shiatsu meridians

Neck
fig. 10.11

Chest
fig. 10.12

Upper arm
fig. 10.15

Upper abdomen
fig. 10.13

Lower arm
fig. 10.16

Lower abdomen
fig. 10.14

Hand
fig. 10.17

Upper leg
fig. 10.18

2004

Fig. 10.4 Posterior lower view: Zen Shiatsu meridians

Upper abdomen
fig. 10.13

Lower abdomen
fig. 10.14

Lower arm
fig. 10.16

Hand
fig. 10.17

Upper leg
fig. 10.18

Lower leg
fig. 10.19

Foot
fig. 10.20

2004

Fig. 10.5 Head anterio-posterior views: Zen Shiatsu meridians

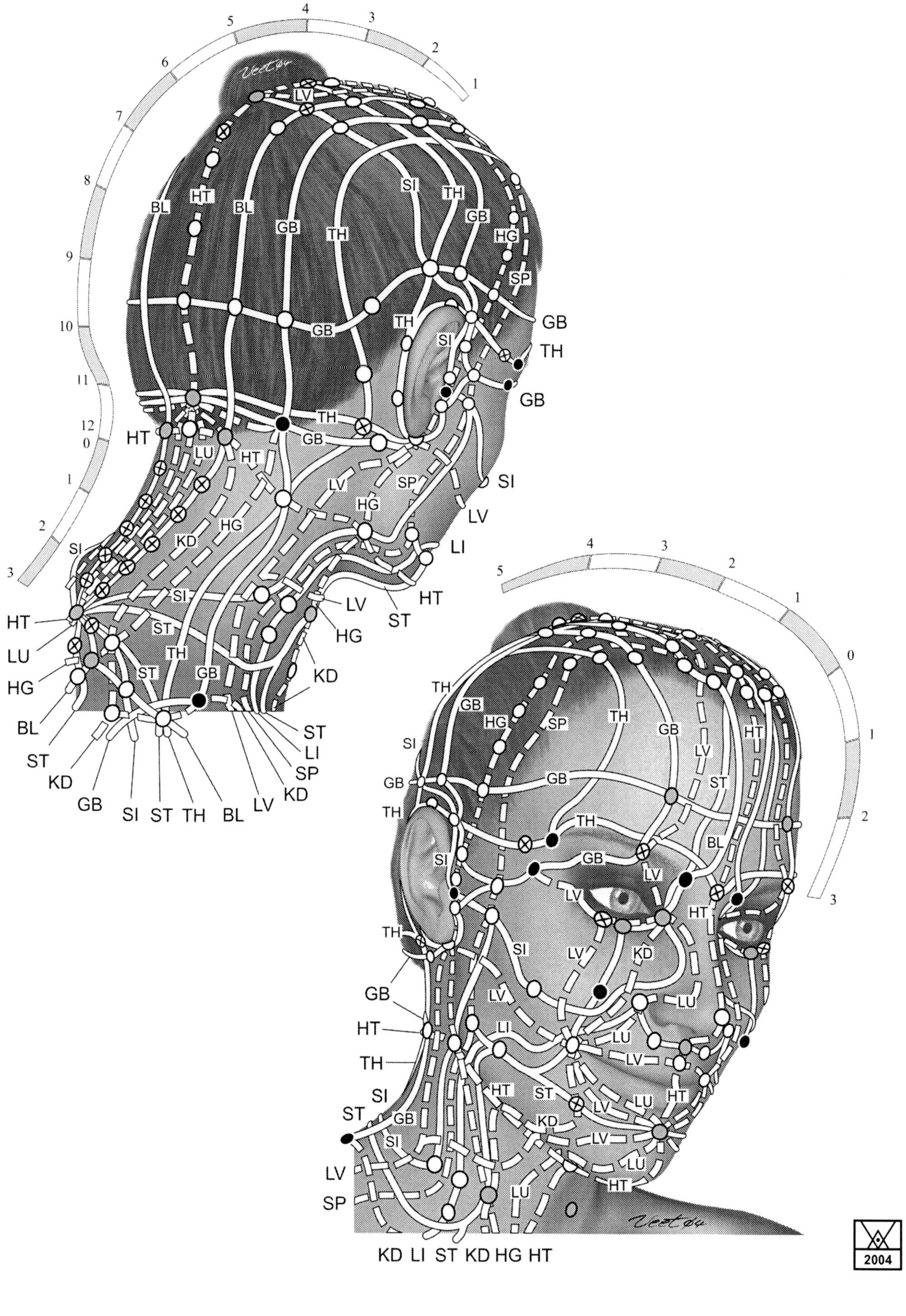

Fig. 10.6 Arm and hand views: Zen Shiatsu meridians

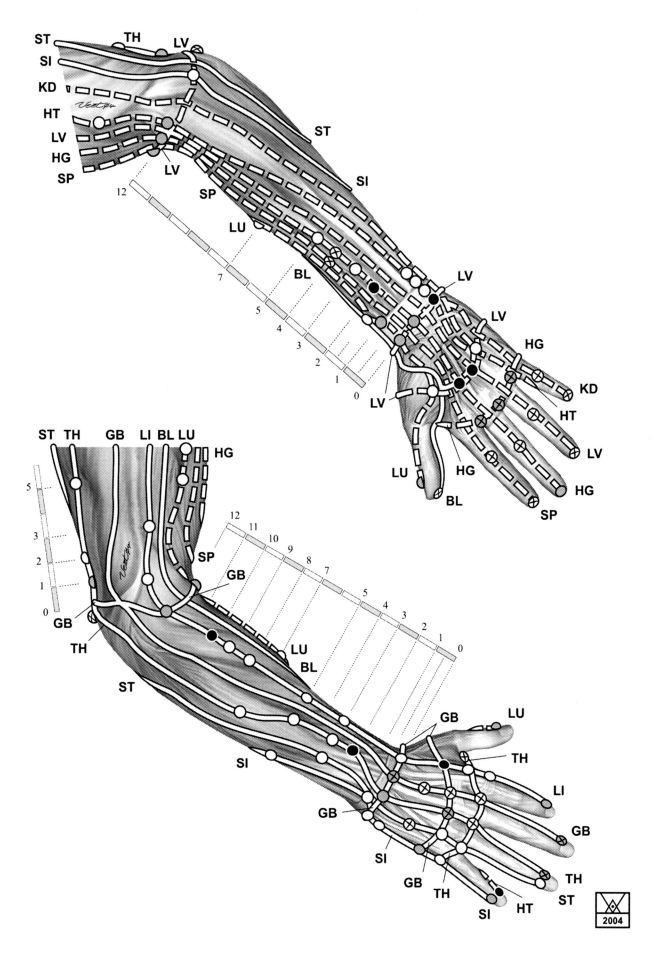

Fig. 10.7 Male perineum: Zen Shiatsu meridians

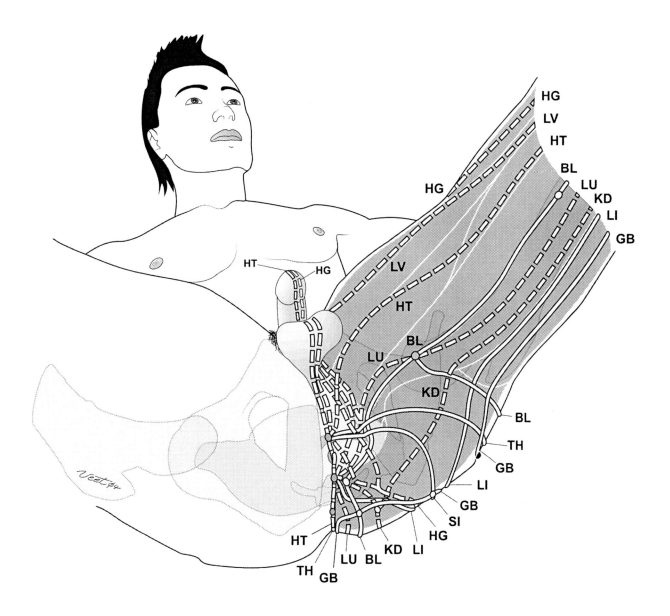

Fig. 10.8 Female perineum: Zen Shiatsu meridians

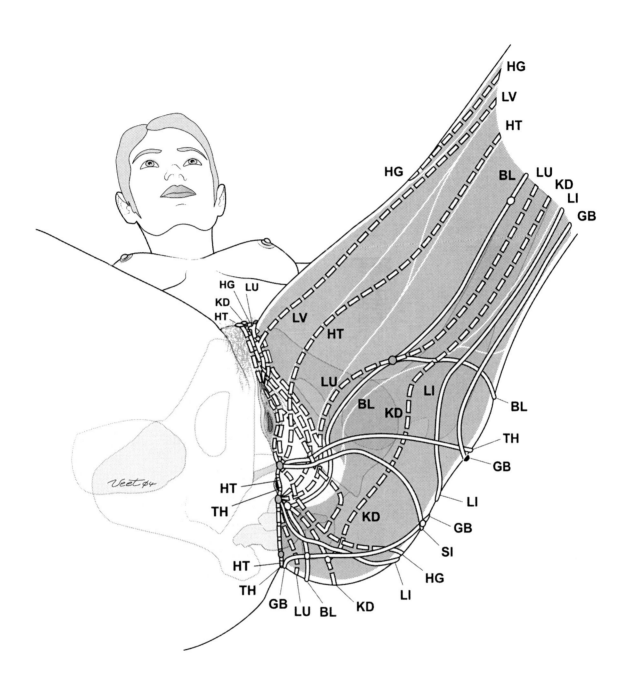

Fig. 10.9 Lower Leg and Foot details: Zen Shiatsu meridians

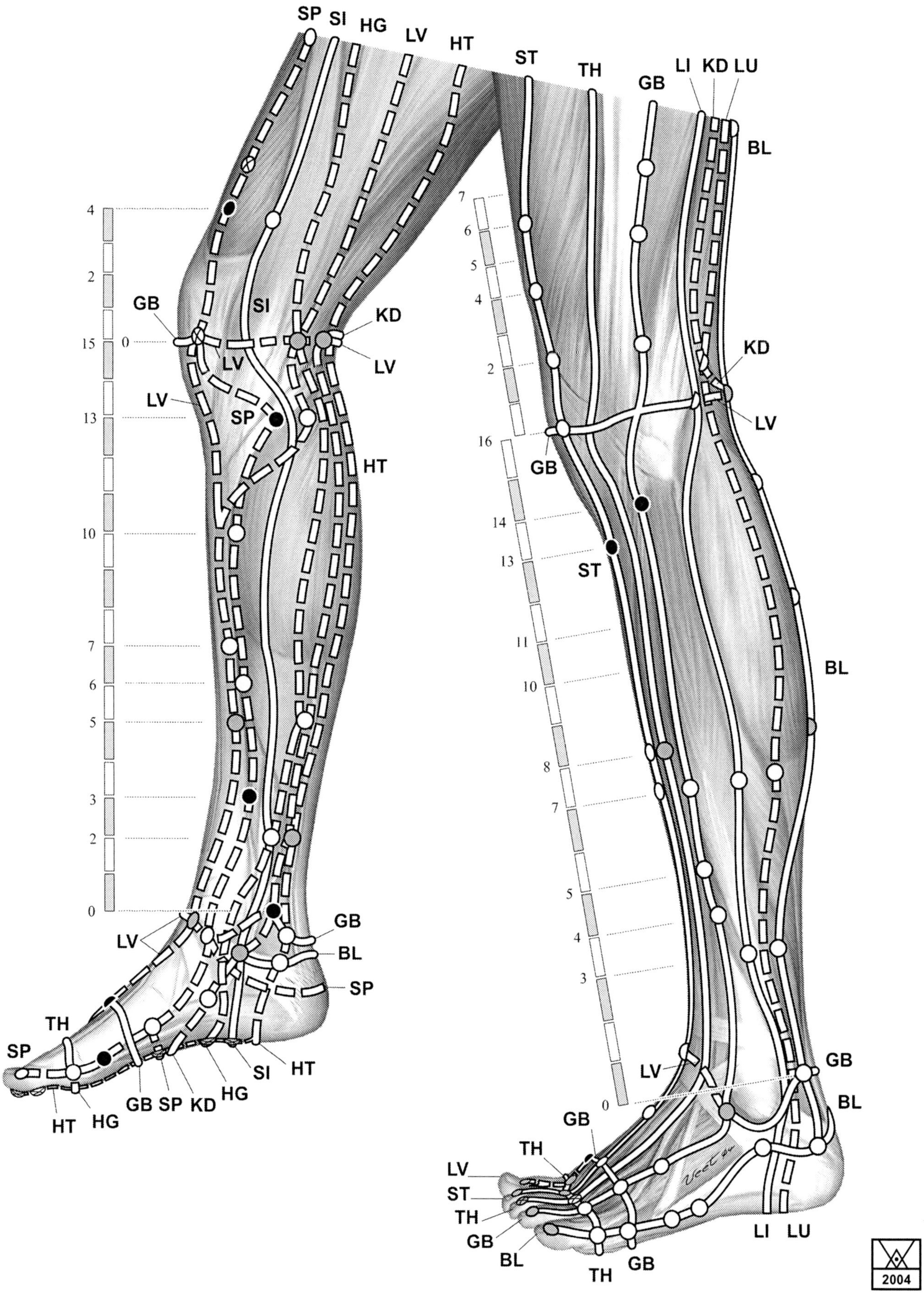

Fig. 10.10 Foot dorsal and plantar details: Zen Shiatsu meridians

Foot: Dorsal view

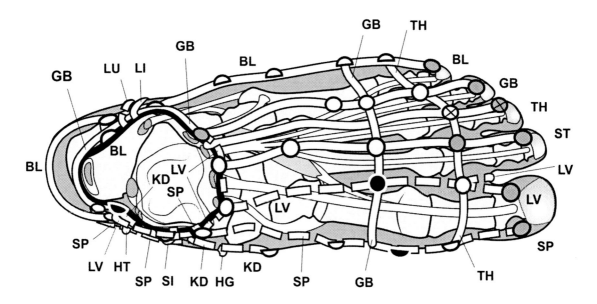

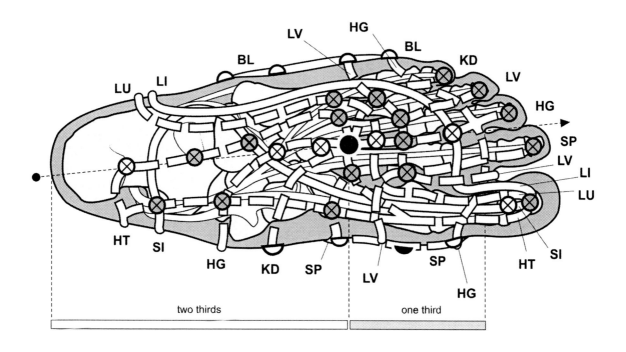

Foot: Plantar view

Fig. 10.11 Cross section through neck at the fifth cervical vertebra

1 Anterior jugular vein
2 Infrahyoid muscles
3 Thyrohyoid membrane
4 Pre-epiglottic fat
5 Epiglottis
6 Cuneiform cartilage
7 Corniculate cartilage
8 Thyroid cartilage
9 External carotid artery
10 Sternocleidomastoid muscle
11 External jugular vein
12 Internal jugular vein
13 Internal carotid artery
14 Scalenus anterior muscle
15 Longus capitas muscle
16 Longus colli muscle

17 Inferior constrictor muscle
18 Phrenic nerve
19 Body of fifth cervical vertebra
20 Vertebral artery within foramen transversarium
21 Scalenus medius muscle
22 Scalenus posterior muscle
23 Spinal cord
24 Levator scapulae muscle
25 Longissimus cervicis muscle
26 Flexor digiti minimi muscle
27 Erector spinae muscle
28 Splenius capitas muscle
29 Trapezius muscle
30 Ligamentum nuchae

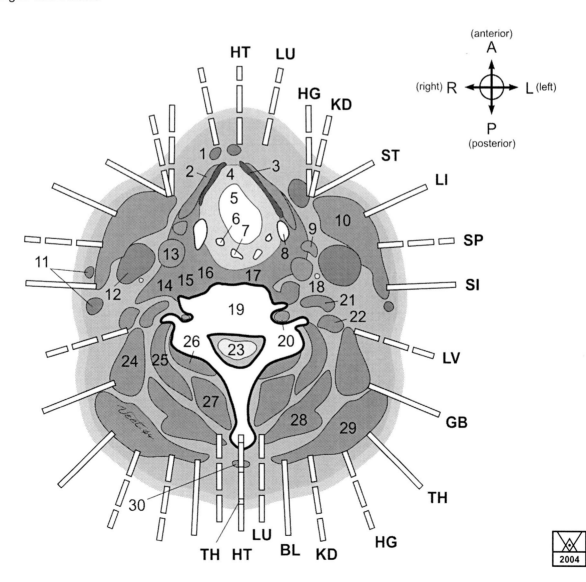

Fig. 10.12 Cross section through chest at the seventh and eigth thoracic vertebra

1 Body of sternum
2 Internal thoracic artery and vein
3 Third costal cartilage
4 Pectoralis muscle
5 Fourth rib
6 Intercostal muscles
7 Fifth rib
8 Serratus anterior muscle
9 Latissimus dorsi muscle
10 Sixth rib
11 Seventh rib
12 Scapula
13 Rhomboidus major muscle
14 Eigth rib
15 Trapezius muscle
16 Erector spinae muscle
17 Spinal cord
18 Intervertebral disc, seventh / eighth
    thoracic vertebra

19 Descending aorta
20 Azygos vein
21 Oesophagus
22 Left bronchus, pulmonary artery and veins
23 Lower lobe of left lung
24 Oblique fissure
25 Upper lobe of left lung
26 Wall of left ventricle
27 Mitrial valve
28 Left atrium
29 Vestibule of left ventrical (to root of aorta)
30 Right ventrical cavity
31 Right auricle (atrial appendage)
32 Right atrium
33 Middle lobe of right lung
34 Oblique fissure
35 Lower lobe of left lung
36 Right bronchus, pulmonary artery and veins

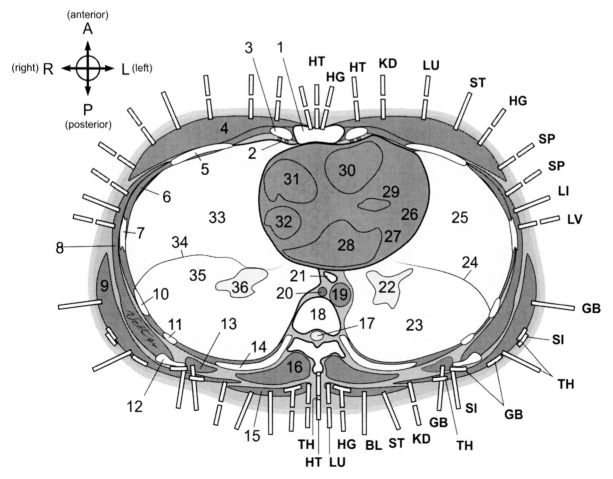

Fig. 10.13 Cross section through upper abdomen at the first lumbar vertebra

1 Stomach body/antrum
2 Head of pancreas
3 First part of duodenum
4 Gall bladder
5 Falciform ligament
6 Rectus abdominis muscle
7 Transverse abdomimis muscle
8 Eighth costal cartilage
9 Latissimus dorsi muscle
10 Ninth costal cartilage
11 External oblique muscle
12 Tenth rib
13 Right lobe of liver
14 Eleventh rib
15 Latissimus muscle
16 Serratus posterior muscle
17 Twelth rib

18 Right kidney
19 Quadratus lumborum muscle
20 Erector spinae muscle
21 Conus medullaris of spinal cord
22 First lumbar vertebra
23 Right crus of diaphragm
24 Inferior vena cava
25 Splenic vein
26 Aorta
27 Left kidney
28 Lower pole of spleen
29 Transverse and descending colon
30 Jejunum
31 Tail of pancreas
32 Left lobe of liver

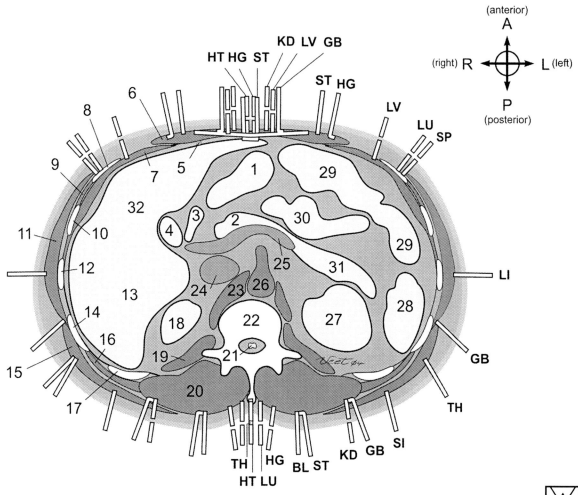

Fig. 10.14 Cross section through lower abdomen at the second sacral segment

1 Linea alba
2 Ileum
3 Mesentery of ileum
4 Greater omentum
5 Caecum
6 Transversus abdominis muscle
7 Internal oblique muscle
8 Axternal oblique muscle
9 Sartorius muscle
10 Gluteus minimis muscle
11 Tensor fasciae latae muscle
12 Gluteus medius muscle
13 Gluteus maximus muscle
14 Ilium and sacral-iliac joint
15 Iliacus muscle
16 Psoas major muscle
17 Right external iliac artery
18 Right external iliac vein

19 Right ureter
20 Right internal iliac vein
21 Right obturator nerve
22 Superior gluteal artery and vein
23 Median sacral artery and vein
24 Second segment of sacrum
25 Filium terminale within sacral canal
26 Second sacral nerve root
27 Right obturator nerve
28 Left external iliac vein
29 Left internal iliac vein
30 Left internal iliac artery
31 Left ureter
32 Left external iliac artery
33 Descending colon
34 Sigmoid colon

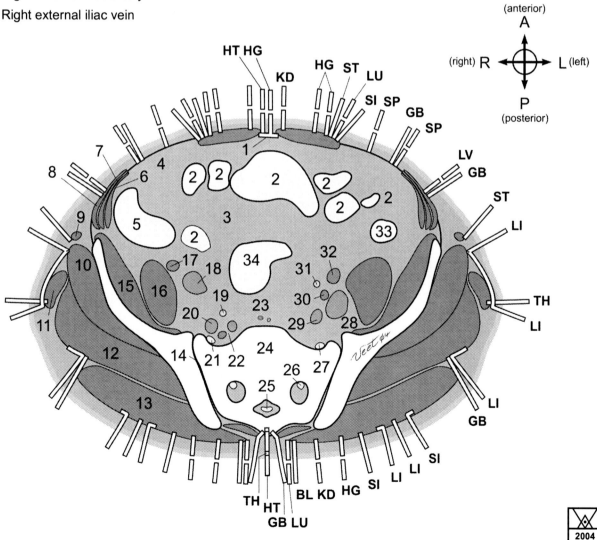

2004

Fig. 10.15 Cross section through arm at the mid-shaft of humerus

1 Biceps brachii muscle
2 Cephalic vein
3 Brachialis muscle
4 Brachioradialis muscle
5 Radial nerve, profunda brachii artery and vein
6 Triceps muscle lateral head
7 Triceps muscle, medial head
8 Triceps muscle, long head
9 Humerus shaft

10 Ulnar nerve
11 Superior ulnar collateral artery and vein
12 Basilic vein
13 Venae comitantes of brachial artery
14 Brachial artery
15 Median nerve
16 Musculocutaneous nerve

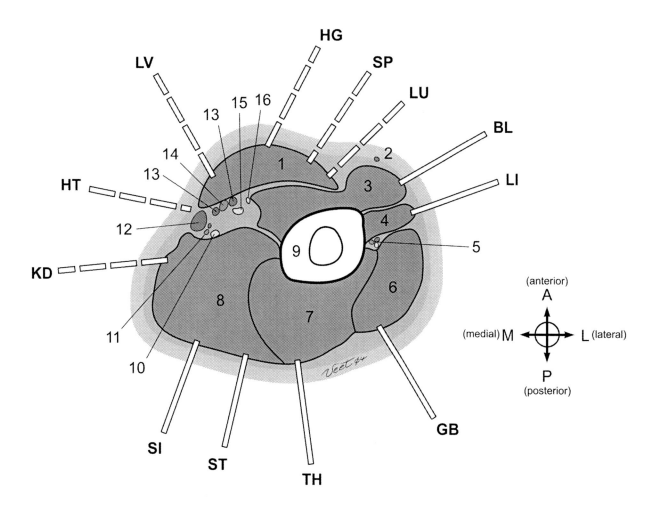

Fig. 10.16 Cross section of lower arm at the elbow inferior to radio-ulnar joint

1 Brachioradialis muscle
2 Cephalic vein
3 Radial artery and venae commitantes
4 Extensor carpi radialis longus muscle
5 Radial nerve
6 Medial recurrent artery and vein
7 Extensor carpi radialis brevis muscle
8 Extensor digitorum muscle
9 Supinator muscle
10 Radius
11 Posterior interosseus artery and vein
12 Extensor carpi unaris muscle
13 Anconeus muscle
14 Ulna

15 Flexor digitorum profundis muscle
16 Posterior recurrent artery and vein
17 Ulnar nerve
18 Flexor carpi ulnaris muscle
19 Flexor digitorum superficialis muscle
20 Brachialis muscle
21 Basilic vein
22 Palmaris longus muscle
23 Flexor carpi radialis muscle
24 Pronator teres muscle
25 Ulnar artery and vein
26 Biceps brachii tendon

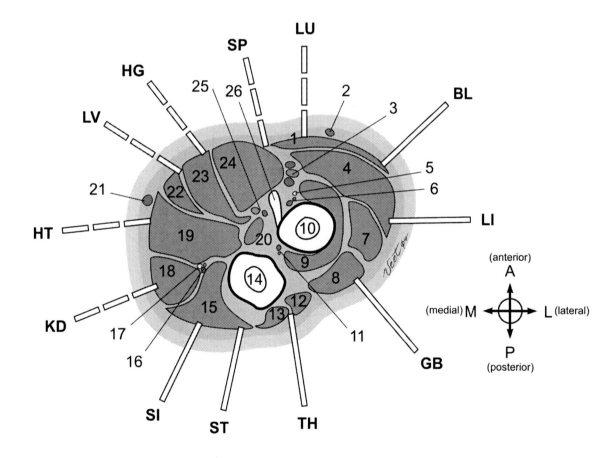

Fig. 10.17 Cross section of hand through the proximal shafts of the metacarpals

1 Palmar aponeurosis
2 Median nerve
3 Flexor pollicis brevis muscle
4 Flexor pollicis longus muscle
5 Abductor pollicis brevis muscle
6 First metacarpal
7 Extensor pollicis brevis tendon
8 Extensor pollicis longus tendon
9 Cephalic vein
10 Radial artery
11 First dorsal interosseus muscle
12 Adductor pollicis muscle
13 Second metacarpal

14 Dorsal and palmar interosseous muscle
15 Extensor indicis tendon
16 Third metacarpal
17 Extensor digitorum tendons
18 Fourth metacarpal
19 Dorsal venous plexus
20 Fifth metacarpal
21 Abductor digiti minimi muscle
22 Opponens digiti minimi muscle
23 Flexor digitorum profundus tendon
24 Flexor digitorum superficialis tendon
25 Ulnar artery and nerve

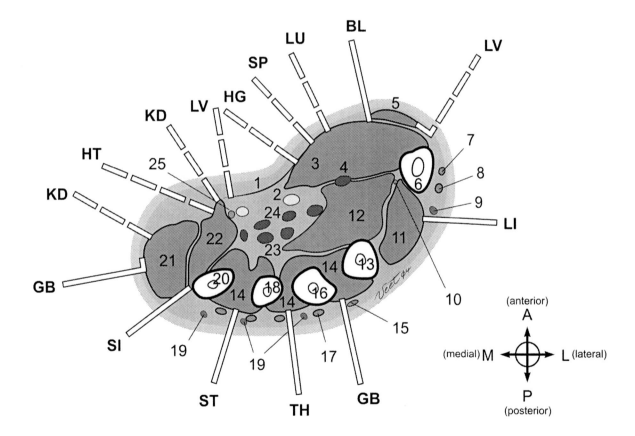

Fig. 10.18 Cross section of upper leg through middle of thigh

1 Vastus lateralis muscle
2 Rectus femoris muscle
3 Vastus medialis muscle
4 Sartorius muscle
5 Vastus intermedius muscle
6 Femoral vein
7 Femoral artery
8 Femur
9 Adductor longus muscle

10 Adductor magnus muscle
11 Gracilis muscle
12 Biceps femoris muscle
13 Sciatic nerve
14 Biceps femoris muscle
15 Semitendinosus muscle
16 Semimembranosus muscle

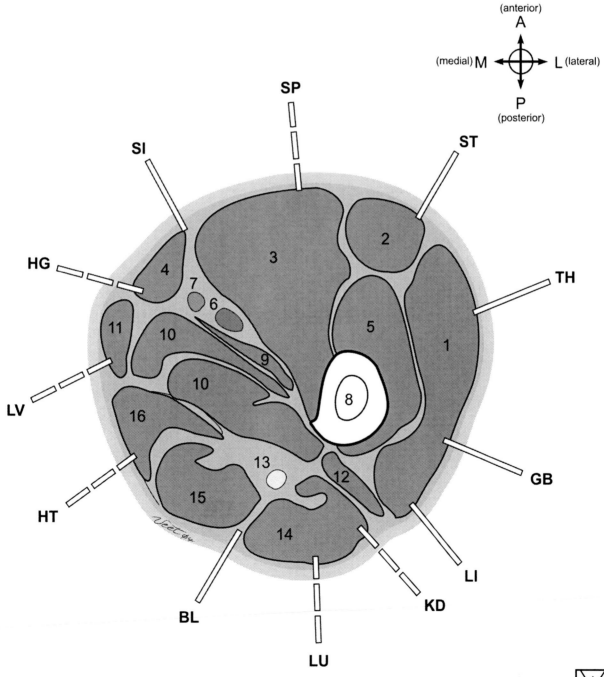

Fig. 10.19 Cross section of lower leg through middle of calf

1 Tibia
2 Tibialis anterior muscle
3 Superficial peroneal nerve
4 Extensor hallucis longus muscle
5 Anterior tibial artery and vein
6 Tibialis posterior muscle
7 Flexor digitorum longus muscle
8 Great saphenous vein
9 Extensor digitorum muscle
10 Peroneus brevis muscle

11 Peroneus longus muscle
12 Fibula
13 Flexor hallucis muscle
14 Peroneal artery with venae commitantes
15 Tibial nerve
16 Tibial artery with venae comitantes
17 Soleus
18 Gastrocnemius muscle (medial head)
19 Gastrocnemius muscle (lateral head)

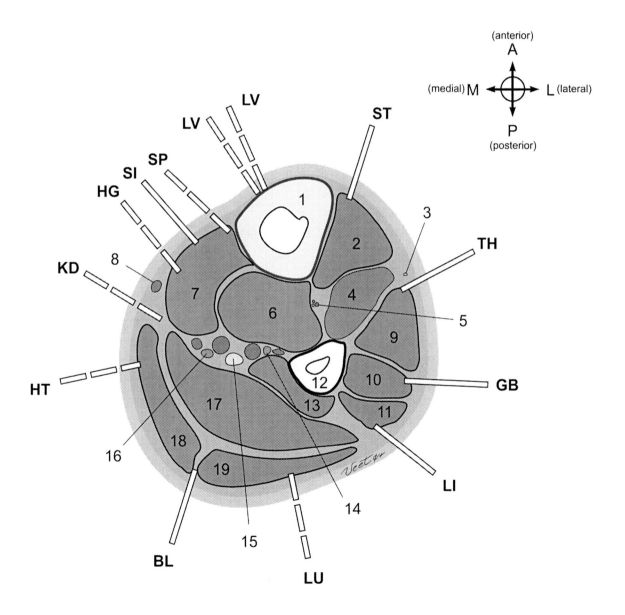

Fig. 10.20 Cross section of foot through bases of the metatarsal bones

1 First metatarsal
2 Second metatarsal
3 Third metatarsal
4 Fourth metatarsal
5 Fifth metatarsal
6 Medial cuneiform
7 Fragment of lateral cunieform
8 Extensor hallucis longus tendon
9 Dorsal pedis artery, vein and nerve
10 Extensor hallucis brevis muscle
11 Extensor digitorum longus tendons
12 Second dorsal metatarsal artey
13 Extensor digitorum brevis muscle
14 Fourth dorsal interosseus

15 Tibialis anterior tendon
16 Medial marginal vein
17 Abductor hallucis muscle
18 Flexor hallucis brevis muscle
19 Flexor hallucis longus tendon
20 Peroneus longus tendon
21 Medial plantar artery, vein and nerve
22 Adductor hallucis (oblique head) muscle
23 Lateral plantar artery, vein and nerve
24 Second plantar interosseus muscle
25 Third plantar interosseus muscle
26 Flexor digiti minimi muscle
27 Opponens digiti minimi muscle
28 Abductor digiti minimi muscle
29 Flexor digitorum longus tendons
30 Flexor digitorum brevis muscle and tendon

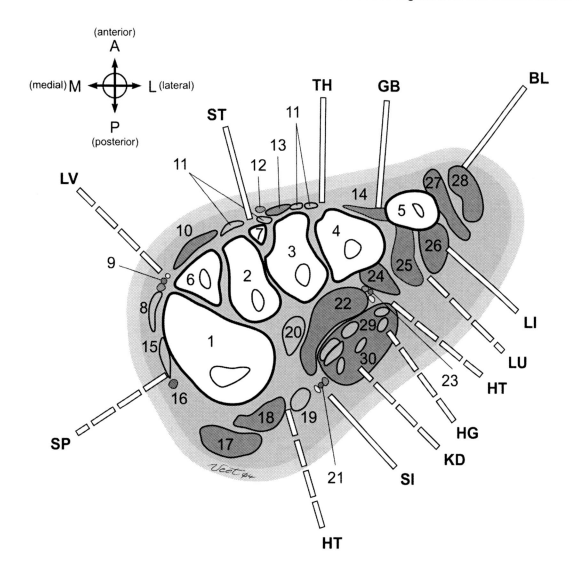

Appendix

Alternative diagnostic illustrations
for
Zen Shiatsu

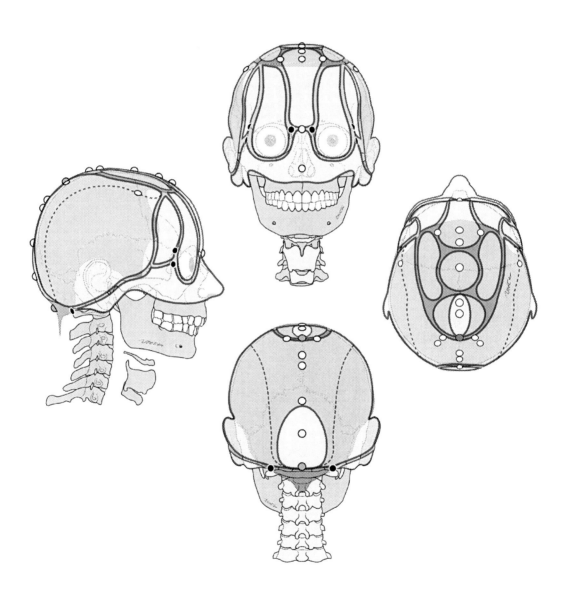

Fig. A.1 Head diagnosis: Top and side views

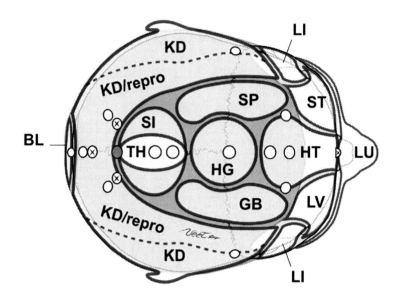

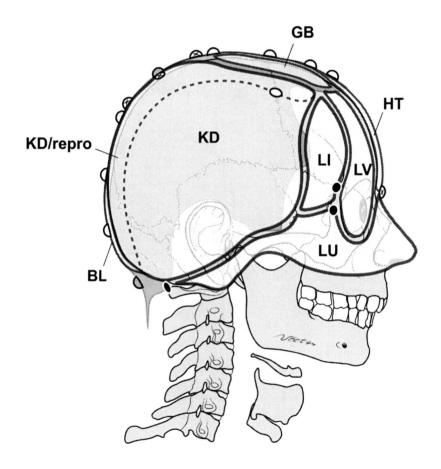

Fig. A.2 Head diagnosis: Front and back views

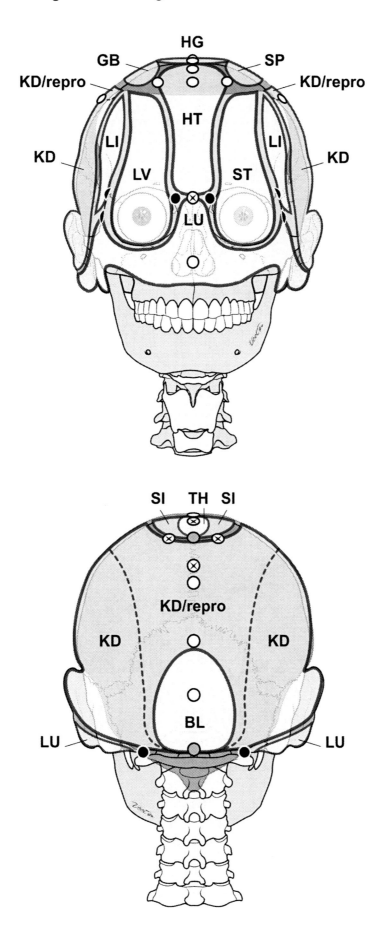

Fig. A.3 Body diagnosis: Back, neck and head

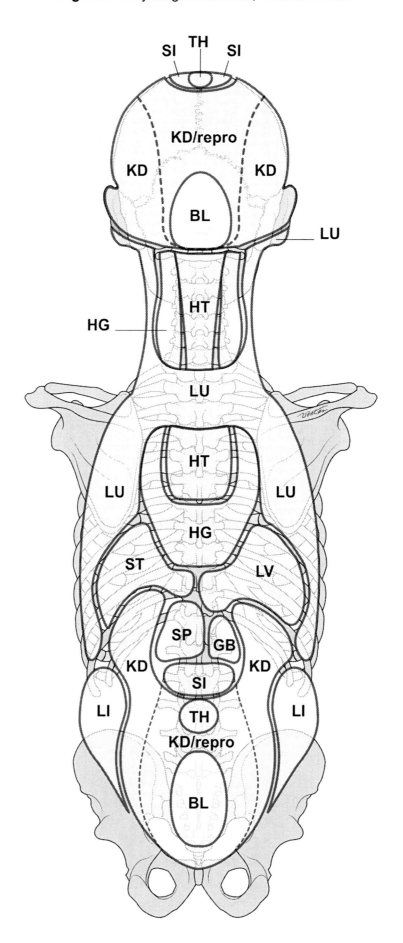

Fig. A.4 Body diagnosis: Hara, neck and head

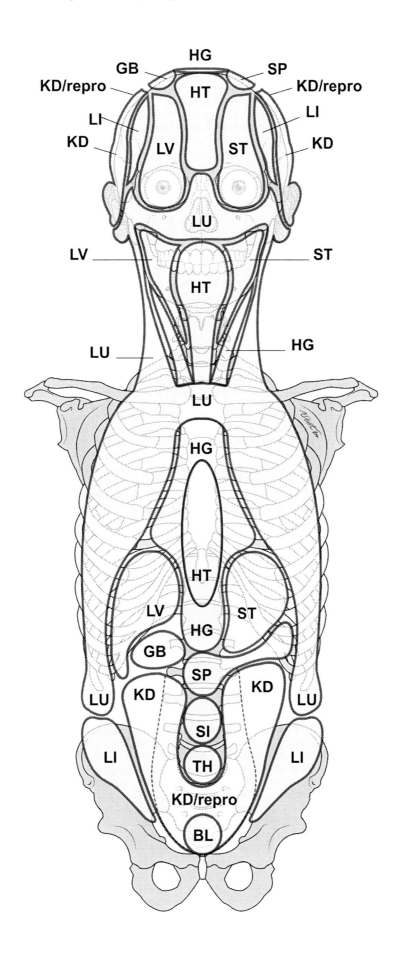

Bibliography

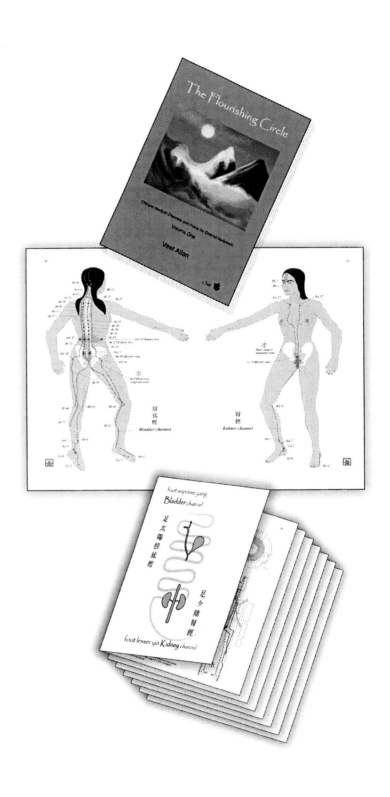

Bibliography

- *A Companion to Medical Studies*
  Vol 1, Anatomy, Biochemistry, Physiology
  and related subjects.
  Passmore, R., Robson, J S (eds)
  Blackwell Scientific Publications,
  Oxford, London, Edinburgh, Melbourne, 1976.

- *A Flourishing Yin*
  Gender in China's Medical History, 960-1665
  Furth, Charlotte
  University of California Press,
  Berkeley, Los Angeles, London, 1999.

- *A Manual of Acupuncture*
  Deadman, Peter., Mazin Al-Khafazi., Kevin Baker
  Journal of Chinese Medicine Publications,
  East Sussex, 1998.

- *Acupuncture Points, Images and Functions*
  Lade, Arnold
  Eastland Press, Seattle, 1989.

- *Anatomy for the Artist*
  Barcsay, Jenő
  Little, Brown and Company, London, 2000.

- *Anatomy of the Living Human*
  Csillag, András
  Könemann Verlagsgesellschaft, Köln, 1999.

- *Anatomy of Movement*
  Calais-Germain, Blandine
  Eastland Press, Seattle, 1993.

- *Bodymind Energetics*
  Towards a Dynamic model of Health
  Seem, Mark
  Thorsons, Wellingborough,1987.

- *Craniosacral Therapy*
  Upledger, John.,Vredevoogd, J.D.
  Eastland Press, Seattle, WA, 1983.

- *Chinese Characters*
  Their origin, etymology, history,
  classification and signification
  Weiger, Dr L (S.J.)
  Dover Publications and Paragon
  Book Reprint Corp,
  New York, 1965

- *Do-In*
  Eastern Massage and Yoga Techniques
  Rofidal, Jean
  Thorsons, Wellingborough, 1981.

- *Extraordinary Vessels*
  Matsumoto, Kiiko., Birch, Steven
  Paradigm Publications, Brookline,
  Massachusetts, 1986.

- *Figure Drawing and Anatomy for the Artist*
  Raynes, John
  Chancellor Press, London, 1993.

- *Fundamentals of Chinese Acupuncture*
  (An Outline of Chinese Acupuncture).
  The Academy of Traditional
  Chinese Medicine, Peking,
  Taraporevala & Sons, Indian edition,
  Bombay, 1988.

- *Hara Diagnosis: Reflections on the Sea*
  Matsumoto, Kiiko., Birch, Steven
  Paradigm Publications, Brookline, 1988.

- *Heart Master and Triple Heater*
  Chinese Medicine from the Classics
  Larre, Claude., Rochat de la Vallée, Elisabeth
  Monkey Press, Cambridge, 1992.

- *Human Cross-Sectional Anatomy*
  Pocket Atlas of body sections and CT Images
  Ellis, Harold., Logan, Bari., Dixon, Adrian.
  Butterworth-Heinnemann, Oxford, 1994.

- *How to see your Health*
  Book of Oriental Diagnosis
  Kushi, Michio
  Japan Publications inc, Tokyo, New York, 1986.

- *Ling Shu or The Spiritual Pivot*
  Translated by Wu Jing-Nuan
  The Taoist Center, Wahington D.C., 2002.

- *Medicine in China*
  A History of Ideas
  Unschuld, Paul U.
  University of California Press
  Berkeley, Los Angeles, London, 1985.

- *Nan-Ching*
  The Classic of Difficulties
  Unschuld, Paul U.
  University of California Press
  Berkeley, Los Angeles, London, 1986.

- *Obstetrics and Gynecology in Chinese Medicine*
  Macioca, Giovanni
  Churchill Livingstone: New York, Edinburgh,
  London, Madrid, Melbourne, San Francisco,
  Tokyo, 1998.

- *Ocean of Streams*
Shiatsu. Meridians, Tsubos and
Theoretical Impressions
Allan, Veet John
Om Shiatsu Centre, Airdrie, 1994.

- *Shiatsu*
Meridian Chart
Masunaga, Shizuto
Iokai Shiatsu Centre, Tokyo, 1970.

- *Shiatsu*
The Complete Guide
Jarmey, Chris., Mojay, Gabriel
Thorsons, London, 1991.

- *Shiatsu Theory and Practice*
A comprehensive text for the student and
professional
Beresford-Cooke, Carola
Churchill Livingstone, 1996.

- *Sotai*
Balance and Health through
Natural Movement
Hashimoto, Keizo .MD with Kawakami, Y
Japan Publications, Tokyo, 1983.

- *Sotai*
Natural Exercise
Hashimoto, Keizo
George Ohsawa Macrobiotic Foundation
Oroville, California, 1981.

- *Spleen and Stomach*
Chinese Medicine from the Classics
Larre, Claude., Rochat de la Vallée, Elisabeth
Monkey Press, Cambridge, 1990.

- *Tao Shiatsu*
Life Medicine for the 21st Century
Endo, Ryokyu
Japan Publications Inc.,Tokyo, New York, 1995

- *The Art of Palpatory Diagnosis
in Oriental Medicine*
Gardner-Abbate, Skya
Churchill Livingstone: Edinburgh, London,
New York,Philadelphia, St Louis,
Sydney, Toronto, 2001.

- *The Book of Shiatsu*
Vitality and health through the art of touch
Lundberg, Paul
Gaia Books Limited, London, 1992

- *The Divinely Responding Classic*
A Translation of the Shen Ying Jing
from the Zhen Jiu Da Cheng
Yang Shou-zhong., Liu Feng-ting
Blue Poppy Press, Boulder, 1994.

- *The Eight Extraordinary Meridians*
Larre, Claude., Rochat de la Valée, Elisabeth
Monkey Press, Cambridge, 1992.

- *The Flourishing Circle*
Chinese Medical Channels and Points
for Oriental Bodywork. Volume One
Allan, Veet
Omki, Thornhill, 2004.

- *The Foundations of Chinese Medicine*
Maciocia, Giovanni
Churchill Livingstone: Edinburgh,
London, Melbourne, New York, 1989.

- *The Heart*
In the Ling shu chapter 8
Chinese Medicine from the Classics
Larre, Claude., Rochat de la Vallée, Elisabeth
Monkey Press, Cambridge, 1991.

- *The Kidneys*
Chinese Medicine from the Classics
Larre, Claude., Rochat de la Vallée, Elisabeth
Monkey Press, Cambridge, 1992.

- *The Liver*
Chinese Medicine from the Classics
Larre, Claude., Rochat de la Vallée, Elisabeth
Monkey Press, Cambridge, 1994.

- *The Lung*
Chinese Medicine from the Classics
Larre, Claude., Rochat de la Vallée, Elisabeth
Monkey Press, Cambridge, 1992.

- *The Macrobiotic Way of Zen Shiatsu*
Sergel, David
Japan Publications inc., Tokyo, New York, 1989.

- *The Newest Illustrations of Acupuncture Points*
Hong Kong: Medicine and Health
Publishing Co, no date.

- *The Numerology of the I Ching*
Huang, Master Alfred
Inner Traditions, Rochester, Vermont, 2000.

- *The Principles of Anatomy and Physiology*
  Seventh edition
  Tortora, Gerard J., Grabowski, Sandra Reynolds
  Harper Collins College Publishers, 1993.

- *The Secret Treatise of the Spiritual Orchard*
  Neijing Suwen Chapter 8
  Chinese Medicine from the Classics
  Larre, Claude., Rochat de la Vallée, Elisabeth
  Monkey Press, Cambridge, 1992.

- *The Shiatsu Workbook*
  A Beginners Guide
  Dawes, Nigel
  Piatkus Books, London, 1991.

- *The Systematic Classic*
  of Acupuncture and Moxibustion
  A Translation of Huang-fu Mi's
  Zhen Jiu Jia Yi Jing
  Yang Shou-Zhong., Chace, Charles
  Blue Poppy Press, Boulder, 1994.

- *The Yellow Emperor's Classic of Internal Medicine*
  Translated by Ilza Veith
  University of California Press, 1972.

- *The Way to Locate Acu-Points*
  Yang Jiasan, Professer (editor)
  Foreign Languages Press, Beijing, 1988.

- *The Web that has no Weaver*
  Kaptchuk, Ted.J.
  Century Hutchinson, London, 1983.

- *Tongue Diagnosis in Chinese Medicine*
  Macioca, Giovanni
  Eastland Press, Seattle, 1987.

- *Tsubo*
  Vital Points for Oriental Therapy.
  Serizawa, Katsusuke
  Japan Publications inc, Tokyo, New York, 1976.

- *Zen Imagery Exercises:*
  Meridian Exercises for Wholesome Living
  Masunaga, Shizuto with Brown, Stephen
  Japan Publications inc., Tokyo, New York, 1987.

- *Zen Shiatsu*
  How to harmonize Yin and Yang for better Health
  Masunaga, Shizuto with Ohashi, Wataru
  Japan Publications inc., Tokyo, New York, 1977.

- *Zen Shiatsu*
  Residential Workshops
  Sasaki, Pauline., Andrews, Clifford
  Grimstone Manor, Horrabridge,
  England, 1989, 1990, 1991.

Glossary of
Chinese Terms

上古天真論篇第一。
昔在黃帝。生而神靈。弱而能言。幼而
徇齊。長而敦敏。成而登天。迺問於天
師曰。余聞上古之人。春秋皆度百歲。
而動作不衰。今時之人。年半百。而動
作皆衰者。時世異耶。人將失之耶。岐
伯對曰。上古之人。其知道者。法於陰
陽。和於術數。食飲有節。起居有常。
不妄作勞。故能形與神俱。而盡終其天
年。度百歲乃去。今時之人不然也。以
酒為漿。以妄為常。醉以入房。以欲
竭其精。以耗散其真。不知持滿。不時
御神。務快其心。逆於生樂。起居無
節。故半百而衰也。夫上古聖人之教
下也。皆謂之虛邪賊風。避之有時。
恬惔虛無。真氣從之。精神內守。病安
從來。是以志閑而少欲。心安而不懼。
形勞而不倦。氣從以順。各從其欲。皆
得所願。故美其食。任其服。樂其俗。
高下不相慕。其民故曰樸。是以嗜欲不
能勞其目。淫邪不能惑其心。愚智賢
不肖。不懼於物。故合於道。所以能年
皆度百歲。而動作不衰者。以其德全不
危也。帝曰。人年老而無子者。材力盡
邪。將天數然也。岐伯曰。女子七歲。
腎氣盛。齒更髮長。二七而天癸至。任
脈通。太衝脈盛。月事以時下。故有
子。三七腎氣平均。故真牙生而長極。
四七筋骨堅。髮長極。身體盛壯。五七
陽明脈衰。面始焦。髮始墮。六七三陽
脈衰於上。面皆焦。髮始白。七七任脈
虛。太衝脈衰少。天癸竭。地道不通。
故形壞而無子也。丈夫八歲。腎氣實。
髮長齒更。二八腎氣盛。天癸至。精氣
溢寫。陰陽和。故能有子。三八腎氣平
均。筋骨勁強。故真牙生而長極。四八
筋骨隆盛。肌肉滿壯。五八腎氣衰。髮
墮齒槁。六八陽氣衰竭於上。面焦。髮
鬢頒白。七八肝氣衰。筋不能動。天癸
竭。精少。腎藏衰。形體皆極。八八則
齒髮去。腎者主水。受五藏六府之精而
藏之。故五藏盛乃能寫。今五藏皆衰。
筋骨解墮。天癸盡矣。故髮白。身體
重。行步不正。而無子耳。帝曰。有其
年已老而有子者。何也。岐伯曰。此其
天壽過度。氣脈常通。而腎氣有餘也。
此雖有子。男不過盡八八。女不過盡七
七。而天地之精氣皆竭矣。帝曰。夫道
者。年皆百數。能有子乎。岐伯曰。夫
道者。能卻老而全形。身年雖壽。能生
子也。黃帝曰。余聞上古有真人者。提
挈天地。把握陰陽。呼吸精氣。獨立守
神。肌肉若一。故能壽敝天地。無有終
時。此其道生。中古之時。有至人者。
淳德全道。和於陰陽。調於四時。去世
離俗。積精全神。游行天地之間。視聽
八達之外。此蓋益其壽命。而強者也。
亦歸於真人。其次有聖人者。處天地
之和。從八風之理。適嗜欲於世俗之
間。無恚嗔之心。行不欲離於世。被服
章。舉不欲觀於俗。外不勞形於事。內
無思想之患。以恬愉為務。以自得為
功。形體不敝。精神不散。亦可以百
數。其次有賢人者。法則天地。象似日
月。辯列星辰。逆從陰陽。分別四時。
將從上古。合同於道。亦可使益壽。
而有極時。

Glossary of Chinese Terms

Vital substances	Body Fluids	津液	*Jin-Ye*
	Blood	血	*Xue*
	Central Qi	中氣	*Zhong Qi*
	Channel Qi	經氣	*Jing Qi*
	Cinnabar Field	丹田	*Dan Tian*
	Corporeal Soul	魄	*Po*
	Defensive Qi	衛氣	*Wei Qi*
	Emperor Fire	君火	*Jun Huo*
	Ethereal Soul	魂	*Hun*
	Essence	精	*Jing*
	Food Qi	谷氣	*Gu Qi*
	Gate of Life	命門	*Ming Men*
	Gathering Qi	宗氣	*Zong Qi*
	Heavenly Gui	天癸	*Tian Gui*
	Intellect/Thought	意	*Yi*
	Minister Fire	相火	*Xiang Huo*
	Nutritive Qi	營氣	*Ying Qi*
	Pre-Heaven Qi	后天之氣	*Hou Tian Zhi Qi*
	Post-Heaven Qi	先天之氣	*Xian Tian Zhi Qi*
	Original/Source Qi	原氣;元氣	*Yuan Qi*
	Spirit-Mind	神	*Shen*
	True Qi	真氣	*Zhen Qi*
	Upright Qi	正氣	*Zheng Qi*
	Will	志	*Zhi*

Channels, vessels and points	Accumulation points	希穴	*Xi Xue*
	Back Transporting points	北俞穴	*Bei Shu Xue*
	Belt Vessel	帶脈	*Dai Mai*
	Bladder channel	膀胱經	*Pang Guang Jing*
	Connecting points	絡穴	*Luo Xue*
	Controller Vessel	任脈	*Ren Mai*
	Extra-ordinary vessels' gathering/confluence points	八脈交會穴	*Ba Mai Jiao Hui Xue*
	Five Transporting points	五俞穴	*Wu Shu Xue*
	Front Collecting points	募穴	*Mu Xue*
	Gathering points	會穴	*Hui Xue*
	Ghost points	鬼穴	*Gui Xue*
	Greater Yang	太陽	*Tai Yang*
	Greater Yin	太陰	*Tai Yin*
	Gall Bladder channel	膽經	*Dan Jing*
	Heart channel	心經	*Xin Jing*
	Heart Governor channel	心主經	*Xin Zhu Jing*
	Kidney channel	腎經	*Shen Jing*
	Large Intestine channel	大腸經	*Da Chang Jing*
	Lesser Yang	少陽	*Shao Yang*
	Lesser Yin	少陰	*Shao Yin*
	Liver channel	肝經	*Gan Jing*
	Lung channel	肺經	*Fei Jing*
	River point	經穴	*Jing Xue*
	Sea point	合穴	*He Xue*
	Small Intestine channel	小腸經	*Xiao Chang Jing*
	Source point	元穴	*Yuan Xue*
	Spleen channel	脾經	*Pi Jing*
	Spring point	熒穴	*Ying Xue*
	Stomach channel	胃經	*Wei Jing*
	Stream point	俞穴	*Shu Xue*

	Supervisor Vessel	督脈	*Du Mai*
	Terminal Yin	厥陰	*Jue Yin*
	Through-way Vessel	衝脈	*Chong Mai*
	Triple Heater channel	三焦經	*San Jiao Jing*
	Well point	井穴	*Jing Xue*
	Yang Brightness	陽明	*Yang Ming*
	Yang Tie Vessel	陽維脈	*Yang Wei Mai*
	Yang Walker Vessel	陽蹻脈	*Yang Qiao Mai*
	Yin Tie Vessel	陰維脈	*Yin Wei Mai*
	Yin Walker Vessel	陰蹻脈	*Yin Qiao Mai*
Five elements	Earth element (movement)	土行	*Tu Xing*
	Fire element	火行	*Huo Xing*
	Metal element	金行	*Jin Xing*
	Water element	水行	*Shui Xing*
	Wood element	木行	*Mu Xing*
	Controlling sequence	相克	*Xiang Ke*
	Generating sequence	相生	*Xiang Sheng*
Pathogenic influences	Cold	寒	*Han*
	Dampness	濕	*Shi*
	Dryness	燥	*Zao*
	Fire	火	*Huo*
	Heat	熱	*Re*
	Pathogenic Qi	邪氣	*Xie*
	Phlegm	痰	*Tan*
	Phlegm-Fluids	痰飲	*Tan Yin*
	Summer Heat	暑	*Shu*
	Wind	風	*Feng*
	Wind-Cold	風寒	*Feng Han*
	Wind-Heat	風熱	*Feng Re*
Emotions (the seven)	Anger	怒	*Nu*
	Fear	恐	*Kong*
	Joy	喜	*Xi*
	Pensiveness	思	*Si*
	Sadness	悲	*Bei*
	Shock	驚	*Jing*
	Worry	憂	*You*
Diagnostic	Abdominal area	腹	*Fu (Hara in Japanese)*
	Atrophy Syndrome	痿征	*Wei Zheng*
	Difficult Urination Syndrome	淋征	*Lin Zheng*
	Empty, Deficiency, or Deplete	虛	*Xu (Kyo in Japanese)*
	Full, Excess, or Replete	實	*Shi (Jitsu in Japanese)*
	Identification of Patterns	辨征	*Bian Zheng*
	Manifestation	標	*Biao*
	Painful Obstruction Syndrome	痹征	*Bi Zheng*
	Point; Tsubo	穴;壷	*Xue; Hu (Tsubo in Japanese)*
	Root	本	*Ben*
	Unit of measurement	寸	*Cun (Sun in Japanese)*
	Wind Stroke	中風	*Zhong Feng*
	Yang Organs	腑	*Fu*
	Yin Organs	臟	*Zang*

Pulse positions	Front pulse location	寸	*Cun*
	Middle pulse location	關	*Guan*
	Rear pulse location	尺	*Chi*
Anatomy	Arm	臂	*Bi*
	Artery	動脈	*Dong Mai*
	Bone	骨	*Gu*
	Brain	腦	*Nao*
	Breast	乳房	*Ru Fang*
	Chest	胸	*Xiong*
	Ear	耳朵	*Er Duo*
	Eyes	眼睛	*Yan Jing*
	Face	面	*Mian*
	Fatty tissue	膏	*Gao*
	Fingers	手指	*Shou Zhi*
	Foot	腳;足	*Jiao; Zu*
	Gall Bladder	膽囊	*Dan Nang*
	Hand	手	*Shou*
	Head	頭	*Tou*
	Heart	心	*Xin*
	Internal Organs	臟腑	*Zang Fu*
	Joint	節	*Jie*
	Knee	膝	*Xi*
	Large Intestine	大腸	*Da Chang*
	Leg	腿	*Tui*
	Liver	肝	*Gan*
	Lung	肺	*Fei*
	Membranes	肓	*Huang*
	Mouth	口	*Ku*
	Muscles	肌肉	*Ji Rou*
	Neck	頸	*Jing*
	Nerve	神經	*Shen Jing*
	Nose	鼻子	*Ba Zi*
	Oesophagus	食管	*Shi Guan*
	Ovary	卵巢	*Luan Chao*
	Pancreas	胰	*Yi*
	Penis	陰莖	*Yin Jing*
	Ribs	肋骨	*Lei Gu*
	Shoulder	肩膀	*Jian Bang*
	Skin	皮肤	*Pi Fu*
	Skeleton	骨骼	*Gu Ge*
	Small Intestine	小腸經	*Xiao Chang*
	Spine	脊椎骨	*Ji Zhui Gu*
	Spinal cord	脊髓	*Ji Sui*
	Spleen	脾	*Pi*
	Stomach	胃	*Wei*
	Tendons	筋	*Jin*
	Testicle	睪丸	*Gao Wan*
	Thigh	大腿	*Da Tui*
	Tongue	舌頭	*She Tou*
	Uterus	子宮	*Zi Gong*
	Vagina	陰道	*Yin Dao*
	Vein	靜脈	*Jing Mai*
	Waist	腰	*Yao*

Point names
and indications Index

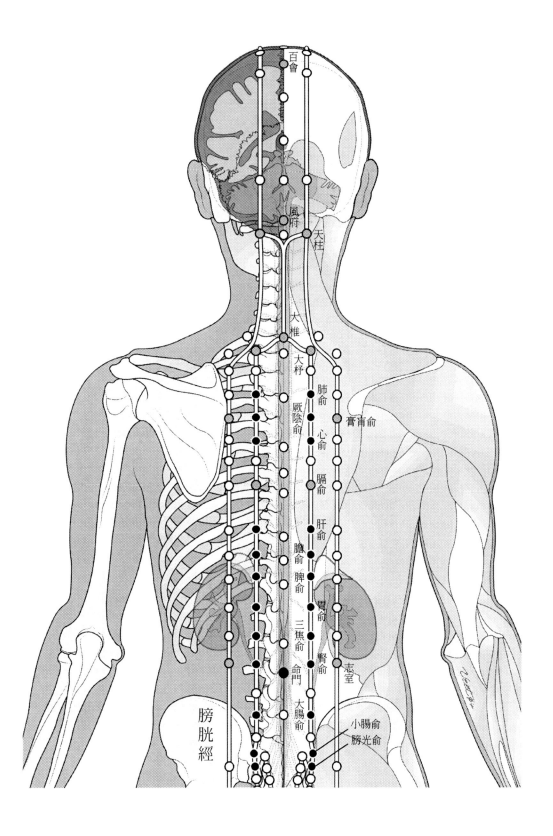

Point names Index

Lung channel 肺經 *Fei-jing*

Large Intestine channel 大腸經 *Da-chang-jing*

Stomach channel 胃經 *Wei-jing*

Spleen channel 脾經 *Pi-jing*

Heart channel 心經 *Xin-jing*

Small Intestine channel 小腸經 *Xiao-chang-jing*

Glossary of extra points illustrated

Head and Neck
Behind the Ball	球後	*Qiuhou*
Beside Container of Fluids	夾承漿	*Jiachengjiang*
Fish Waist	魚腰	*Yuyao*
Four Spirit Hearing	四神聰	*Sishencong*
Nose Passage	鼻通	*Bitong*
Peaceful Sleep	安眠	*Anmian*
Seal Hall	印堂	*Yintang*
Supreme Yang	太陽	*Taiyang*

Chest and Abdomen
Lift with Support	提托	*Tituo*
Three Moxibustion	三角灸	*Sanjiaojiu*
Uterus	子宮	*Zigong*

Back and Waist
Below 17th Vertebra	十七椎下	*Shiqizhuixia*
Hua Tuo's Paravertebral points	華佗夾脊	*Huatuojiaji*
Pacify Asthma	定喘	*Dingchuan*
Stomach Controller Lower Shu	胃管下俞	*Ganshu*
Waist's Eyes	腰眼	*Yaoyan*

Arm
Elbow Tip	肘尖	*Zhoujian*
Front of Shoulder	肩前	*Jianqian*
Two Whites	二白	*Erbai*

Hand
Eight Evils	八邪	*Baxie*
Four Seams	四縫	*Sifeng*
Lumbar Pain Point	要痛穴	*Yaotongxue*
Stiff Neck	落枕	*Luozhen*
Ten Drainings	十宣	*Shixuan*

Leg
Appendix Point	闌尾穴	*Lanweixue*
Crane's Peak	鶴頂	*Heding*
Gall Bladder Point	膽囊穴	*Dannangxue*
Hundred Insect's Den	百蟲窩	*Baichongwo*
Knee Eyes	膝眼	*Xiyan*

Foot
Big Toe's Tranverse Crease	拇趾橫紋	*Muzhihengwen*
Eight Winds	八風	*Bafeng*
Foot's Centre	足心	*Zuxin*
Front and Back's Hidden Pearls	前後陰珠	*Qianhouyinzhu*
Inside Inner Courtyard (ST-44)	里內廷	*Lineiting*
Lost Sleep	失眠	*Shimian*

Point indications Index   ** page numbers are in brackets**

the oriental medical books and illustrations by veet allan

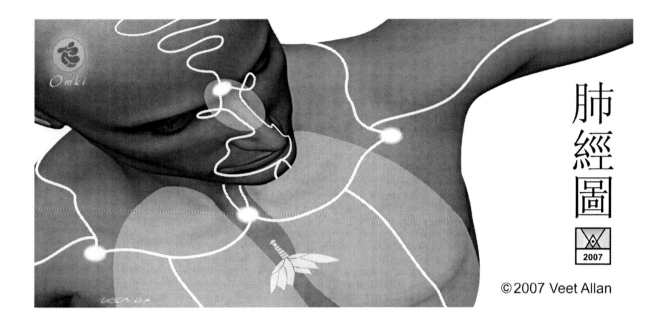

肺經圖

2007

© 2007 Veet Allan

Please visit the Omki website at

www.omki.co.uk

for the latest information on

all publications

including errata, updates and downloads

Lightning Source UK Ltd.
Milton Keynes UK
UKOW012326031212

203137UK00012B/632/A